Holistic Healing

and the
Edgar Cayce Readings

BOOKS BY THE AUTHOR

PSYCHIC MAGIC
1998: THE YEAR OF DESTINY Book 1
1998: THE YEAR OF DESTINY Book 2
HOLISTIC HEALING and the EDGAR CAYCE READINGS

Holistic Healing

and the
Edgar Cayce Readings

RAYMOND OUELLETTE

AERO PRESS PUBLISHERS

P. O. Box 2091   Fall River, Massachusetts 02722

Library of Congress Catalog Card Number: 80-80446

ISBN-0-936450-07-X

Printed in the United States of America

This book is humbly dedicated to the understanding of the philosophy of body, mind, and spirit, and to the attunement of consciousness to that level of awareness that HOLISTIC HEALING may manifest within and without.

"For, in each physical organism there are those conditions that enable the organ to reproduce itself, if it has the co-operation of every other portion of the body. When these suffer from mental or physical disorders that make for repressions in any portion of the system, then first dis-ease and distress arise. If heed is not taken as to the warnings sent forth along the nervous systems of the body indicating that certain organs or portions of the system are in distress, or the S.O.S. call that goes out is not heeded, then disease sets in."

Edgar Cayce reading # 531-2

"Remember, the whole body--physically, mentally, spiritually--is one; and it is as each portion of the system coordinates with the other that there is the better attaining of the normal balance and activity."

Edgar Cayce reading # 920-13

"But if the body is fed only upon that which is temporal in its concept, in its activity, then it MUST of itself become a burden sooner or later."

Edgar Cayce reading # 1691-1

TABLE OF CONTENTS

Nature comes to the succor of the deserted;
when all is lacking she gives back her self.
She flourishes and grows green amidst ruins;
she has ivy for the stones and love for man.

Victor Hugo

FOREWORD

Every person who possesses this book should become related to it in one of two ways:
1. Either as a reader
2. Or as a student

Only the latter will accomplish the full results of the work. There are three things to do:
1. To study
2. To think
3. To execute

There can be such a thing as reading that which is deep and student-like; but a casual reader, who absorbs nothing, is the most superficial of all persons. Whoever reads the fewest books is apt to be the best thinker. A rapid reader cannot be a student.

A casual reading of this book will produce in the pupil no results whatsoever. It will be time wasted; but perhaps well wasted.

The author prefers that no person should have the custody of this book, excepting the owner, or excepting the person who is to use it. A book of study should have but one owner.

Lending and borrowing are relics of barbarism, and twin brothers of poverty and bad business methods.

Polonius, in Hamlet says:

"Neither a borrower nor a lender be;
For loan oft loses both itself and friend.
And borrowing dulls the edge of husbandry."

But a stronger reason prevails in the present instance. The purchaser of this book, or whoever studies it, should at once procure a writing pad or booklet and keep a diary or a record of notes of the experiences relating to the material being learned, applied, and of their results. Annotations of all kinds appertaining to the study and practice will in time be found most beneficial and of great value to the student of this volume.

The high character of the results to be attained
necessitates constant companionship of book and user,
which is impossible if two friends or two members of
the same family are using the same copy; and is just
as inconvenient as one plate would be if two hungry
people were eating out of it.

The mark of a true student is in note-making.
People who absorb the most, observe the most; and the
noteworthy facts are preserved. This has been true of
every successful man and woman who has ever lived;
and a thousand instances might be cited of those who
preserved in the form of notes, every occurrence and
experience that had any value.

There is an axiom that there is no limit to the
powers and capabilities of man when directed by Mind
and Will. A human being unlike an animal is capable of
anything on the physical, the mental and the spiritual planes.

Perfection is available to all, if one is but
willing to pay the price. Happy learning.

INTRODUCTION

There are two principal methods of keeping our health over the encroachment of disease. One is the combative, the other, preventative. The trend of modern medical research and practice in our great colleges and endowed research institutes is almost entirely along combative lines, while the individual, progressive physician learns to work more and more along preventative lines. The slogan of modern medical science is, "Kill the germ and cure the disease." The usual procedure is to wait until acute or chronic diseases have fully developed and then, if possible, to subdue them by means of drugs, by surgical operations, and by means of the morbid products of further disease in the form of serums, antitoxins, vaccines, etc. The combative method fights disease with disease, poison with poison, and germs with germs and germ products. In the language of the Good Book, it is "Bellzebub against the devil."

The preventative method does not wait until the disease has fully developed and gained the ascendancy in the body, but concentrates its best endeavors on preventing, by hygienic living and by natural methods of treatment, the development of diseases. By these it endeavors to put the human body in such a normal, healthy condition that it is practically foolproof against infection or contagion by any disease taints and miasms, and against the inroads of germs, bacteria, and parasites.

The question is, which is the most practical, the most successful and most popular? Which will stand the test of "the survival of the fittest," in the great struggle for existence.

The medical profession has good reason to be alarmed by the inroads made in its work by irregular, unorthodox systems, schools and cults of treating

11

human ailments; but instead of raging at the audacious presumptions of these interlopers, would it not be much better to inquire if there is not some reasons for the astonishing results causing the spread and popularity of such therapeutic innovations?

Their success undoubtedly is based on the fact that they concentrate their best efforts on preventive instead of combative methods of treating disease. People are beginning to realize that it is cheaper and more advantageous to prevent disease than it is to cure it. To create and maintain continuous, buoyant good health means greater efficiency for physical and mental work; greater capacity for the true enjoyment of life, and the best insurance against failure and poverty because of decimated health. Therefore, he who builds constructive and progressive health is of greater value to humanity than he who allows himself to drift into the destructive aspects of disease through ignorance of the laws of nature, and attempts to cure himself by doubtful and uncertain combative methods.

It is said that in China the physician is hired and paid by the year; and that he receives a certain stipend as long as the members of the family stay in good health, but that the salary is suspended as long as one of his charges is ill. If some similar method of engaging and paying for medical services were in vogue in this country the trend of medical research and practice would soon undergo a radical change of no mean consequence.

The dietetic expert, the hydropath, the physical culturist, the osteopath, the mental and spiritual healer, and the Christian Scientist, do not pay much attention to the pathological conditions or to the symptoms of disease. They regulate the diet and habits of living on a natural basis, promote elimination, and teach correct breathing and systematic exercises, correct mechanical lesions of the spine, establish the right and emotional attitude and, in so far as they succeed in doing this, they build health and therefore diminish the possibility of disease. The successful doctor of the future will have to fall in line with the procession of these natural systems, and do more teaching than prescribing.

I realize that many of the statements and claims made in this volume will seem radical and irrational to many individuals and to the established school of thought regarding regular medicine. They will say that most of the teachings herein are actually contrary to the firmly established theories of medical science. However, let us not judge too hastily; to observe, to think and to test, and I am certain that they will verify this by their own actual experiences with "HOLISTIC HEALING." Medical science has had to abandon in the past innumerable theories and practices which at one time or another were as firmly established as some of the pet theories of the present day.

None of the statements made in this volume are meant to deny the necessity of combative methods under certain circumstances. What we wish to emphasize is that the regular school of medicine is spending much too much of, its efforts along combative lines, and not enough along preventative applications. It would be foolish to deny the necessity of surgery in traumatism, and in abnormal conditions requiring mechanical means of adjustment or treatment.

Such necessity, as for instance, will exist in certain obstetrical cases, as long as women have not learned, or are not willing to live in such a way as to make surgical intervention unnecessary in childbirth. As long as people persist in violating the laws of their being, and thereby make their bodies prolific breeding grounds for disease taints, germs and parasites, which are bound to provoke inflammatory, feverish processes, combative measures will have to be resorted to by the physician. So precautionary measures against infection will have to be observed, and these should be in harmony with nature's endeavors, not contrary and suppressive; they should tend to conserve and not to destroy.

Natural dietetics, fasting, hydrotherapy, osteopathy, chiropractic, and mental therapeutics, are combative as well as preventative, but if properly applied they do not in any way injure the organism or interfere with nature's intent and its natural methods. This cannot be said for much of the surgical and medical treatment of the old school of medicine. We criticize and condemn only those methods which are suppressive and destructive rather than curative.

In many instances the warnings and teachings of natural living and health have already been verified, and will have to be heeded and accepted by medical science at the insistence of the majority of the people, who have to this day been so cruelly exploited by an insensitive medical profession.

It is not the purpose or the intention of this book to diagnose or prescribe for any specific ailment; this is merely a compilation of the author's findings from his research of the Edgar Cayce readings on subjects related to HOLISTIC HEALING. It must be borne in mind at all times that the recommendations enumerated in this study were recommended for specific individuals, and although the suggestions and formulas comprises only items which may be obtained without a prescription, responsibility for any and all attempts to research and apply such suggestions and formulas as reported herein must lie with the reader alone.

CHAPTER ONE

INITIATION

When I became acquainted with the psychic readings of the Edgar Cayce legacy, one of the very first impressions I received from their perusal, was the perfect parallel between its teachings and the schools of natural healing and cures.

I saw at once that the same laws and principles which constitute the basis of the Holy Book, on the ethical, moral and spiritual planes of being, also control the processes of health, dis-ease and cure, on the physical and mental planes. In other words, it became apparent to me that the harmony of the ethical and moral law, have their perfect correspondence in the constitution of the physical body, and its co-related physical, mental and emotional activities.

"As for the physical body, this is made up of the elements of the various natures that keep same in its motion necessary for sustaining its equilibrium; as begun from its (the individual's body) first cause." 281-24

In our halcyon days of youthful vigor, we are apt to look upon health culture, mind training, and higher philosophy with contempt and derision; but suffering is the great awakener, revealer and teacher, as proven by the ones seeking healing from Cayce and obtaining it in most cases, even though most were given up as incurable by the medical profession. So long as we are prosperous, and suffering does not overtake us, we are content to jog along in the old ruts, and to live in "the good old ways" to the very limit of nature's endurance.

I had learned the ten commandments, but neither in church, nor school, had I been taught there exist a decalogue and a morality of the physical, as well as of the spiritual. I had been left in absolute ignorance of the laws of nature and of my own being. Following the example of friends and boon companions, I imagined that the highest philosophy of life was to "have a good time while it lasted," and "let tomorrow take care of itself."

In church I was taught that confession followed with repentance would insure the forgiveness of my sins, and the salvation of my soul.

I accepted the popular belief that life and death, health and dis-ease, are largely a matter of chance, dependent upon drafts, wet feet, germs and viruses, and upon the inscrutable will of a capricious Providence, to say the least.

My good friends, as well as the doctors, assured me that eating and drinking and the use of tobacco and alcohol, had very little to do with man's physical condition. They said to me: "Eat and drink what agrees with you (that is, what tastes good and makes you feel good); satisfy your physical appetites and cravings to the fullest extent, as it is only natural to do so. If you should therefore get into any trouble, come to us and we will fix you up all right again." Once more, the comfortable doctrines of, "Do as you please," and of "Vicarious salvation," arises.

I now know that such advice is still administered constantly and promiscuously to the youth not only of our country but of the world, in private consultations, in open clinics, and by physicians of good repute.

Neither was the trend of this popular philosophy conducive to the strenghtening of my moral fiber and character.

Leaders of modern thought, many of them highly respected college professors and renowned scientists, boldly applied the speculation of the evolutionary theories to the origin and development of religion, of ethics and of morality.

According to their teachings mental and emotional activities are chemical reactions of physical brain and nerve matter; there have been all kinds of forces existent in history, except ethical forces; so ethics and morality grow out of customs, and are not antecedent to them; moral standards are all a matter of evolution, custom and expediency, and are subject to changes, like fashions in woman's hats and dresses. So, ethical and moral notions are mere figments of speculation and imagined realities, which should be discarded, the sooner the better.

"Common sense" business men told me that their highest ethical principle was: "Do to the other fellow, lest he do to you." This is in direct contradiction of that given in the Holy Book and the readings of Edgar Cayce as so stated in the following.

"For 'As ye would that men should do to you, do ye even so to them' is not merely an axiom but a life, an experience, a consciousness, that may bring the greater bulwark of safety under any condition or experience that may be practiced in the experiences of a soul or entity." 1468-1

As a result of all these false teachings and examples of personal irresponsibility and of ethical and moral nihilism, chaos filled my mind and soul. I did not know what to believe, nor what to disbelieve and as a natural result, I did not care how I lived; my only concern was the gratification of my physical appetites and of my desire for diversion and amusement.

The first part of my life, up to the age of manly maturity was a sort of experiment to see how far and how long I could go on in the violation of the rules of wholesome living, without suffering immediately, and drastically, nature's penalties.

Finally, however, I reached the limits of nature's endurance, and I began to suffer greatly from the natural results of my ignorance and foolishness.

Following the advice of my friends, the doctors, I sought relief and cure with drugs. I consulted many physicians but their pills and potions, at best, only gave temporary relief. At the age of forty, I was a physical and mental wreck. I had lost all faith in God, in Nature and in myself. So many times I had to fight a strong desire to end my misery by suicide.

The terror of it all was the utter ignorance and helplessness in which I thereby found myself. I failed
to see clearly the causes of my emotional and mental
troubles, much less the way out of them. However, the
darkest hours are those just before the dawn.

CHAPTER TWO

THE UNITY OF DISEASE AND CURE

One day while walking along Main Street detesting my deplorable condition, I walked unintentionally into the local book store. Of all the books there on display I chanced upon "THE SLEEPING PROPHET." This book by its quick perusal I felt might do me some good. So I, therefore, bought it. It was one of the very first biographies published on the life of Edgar Cayce and of his selfless devotion to people in need of help. This book was written by Jess Stearn, a newspaper reporter, and a new pioneer investigator and writer of the psychic dimension. Written in simple language, and convincing reasoning, it has brought out the fact that Edgar Cayce while asleep, or in trance on his couch could diagnose the ailments of anyone by simply giving him the name and location of the person seeking the reading.

These trance readings given by Cayce and recorded by a stenographer stated that all diseases, barring accidents and surroundings hostile to human life, is due to our violation of nature's laws, and to our common erroneous habits of living; and that, therefore, the fundamental principle of true healing--physically, mentally and spiritually--must consist of the return to natural habits of living and of proper thinking. He stated very simply that we are what we eat as well as what we think.

> *"For what we think and what we eat--combined together--make what we are, physically and mentally." 288-38*

His readings demonstrate the unity of disease and cure, showing that all diseases, in the final analysis, is due to disobedience of natural laws antecedent to the primary effect, namely, the accumulation

19

of effete matter and poisons in the organism; that,
this morbid soil is the breeder of germs and viruses,
and that waste matter clogging the cells and tissues
of the body, becomes the cause of lowered vitality
by obstructing the flow of blood and nerve currents,
and by hindering the vibratory activities of the cells
and the glands of the endocrine system of the body.
From these premises it is reasoned that the primary
principle of true healing must be in the elimination
of waste and foreign matter from the system, through
natural methods of living and thinking; that poisoning
and mutilating the human organism cannot be conducive
to good health.

> "There is only that necessary, for the full
> physical normal condition, to keep the mind
> and the body active, and to keep the elimina-
> tions near normal. This is, as we find, nec-
> essary in every physical being." 1653-3

> "...there are many channels through which
> eliminations are carried on. First, in the
> respiratory system. This not merely the deox-
> idization being thrown off through the breath,
> or through the clarifications of the blood-
> stream as it flows to the lungs for the oxygen
> necessary to carry on certain conditions...
> but also that of the whole of the exterior...
> through the various pores of the system (and
> that of the lymphatic circulation.)" 5439-1

Also:

> "Keep the eliminations in the system acting
> normally and properly, even though enemas and
> cleansing of the colon is resorted to--which
> is well for anyone to do, for through same
> many reinfections take place by overtaxing
> the system with drosses from fermentation as
> takes place in ascending or traverse (trans-
> verse)? colon." 5717-1

When I read the book, "THE SLEEPING PROPHET," it seemed as though a great light was rising before me and illuminating my darkened consciousness. For the first time in my life I realized that the processes of life and death, of health, disease and cure, were subject to the workings of natural laws, as definite and exact as the laws of gravitation and of chemical affinity; that there was a decalogue and a morality of the physical as well as the mental and spiritual, and that, if I faithfully complied with the laws of my physical nature, there was hope of regeneration rather than degeneration, and the recovery of health, physically, emotionally and mentally. I read engrossed through the night and into the early morning hours, until I had absorbed the contents of the book; and the very next morning, in the bathroom and at breakfast, I began the practice of the natural regime, and carried it out from that time on to the best of my ability.

The results were most gratifying. There were ups and downs and healing crises, but all along, to my great joy, I noticed steady improvement in all of my symptoms. The satisfaction and happiness this gave me were indescriable. They were caused not only by the general improvement in health but by the consciousness that I was working out my own salvation through this newly acquired knowledge along with and by my own personal efforts. Joyfully I realized that I finally had arisen out of utter ignorance and helplessness, and had become independent of the quackery of false philosophy, ignorant priestcraft, and faulty medicine; that I was from that time on the master of my own fate.

I had at last sensed the great fundamental fact of human life and action. That knowledge of natural laws, and the conscious and voluntary co-operation with these laws, is the master key leading to the higher development of man above the purely animal plane of being; and that on the same basis of truth and law only, can the human race at large work out its vaster and more complex problems.

I recognized the unity of disease and cure as applicable not only in the physical body, but also in

the mental and spiritual body. I saw that in the final
analysis, all that we call sin, disease, suffering or
evil, is identical in origin and nature as is healing;
that all of these abnormal and undesirable conditions
are due only to violations of nature's laws and that
therefore the only possible, permanent cure can only be
the result of a return to nature, and living in compliance with her basic fundamental laws and principles.

*"Now as for this entity, and how he may apply
the truth, the law and the knowledge of a
physical-material nature, of dietetics and the
like. We have already indicated that certain
tendencies and weaknesses are present in the
body. They are not diseases--rather dis-eases,
when certain stresses or strains are brought
to bear in the mental, in the spiritual and in
the physical experience of the entity." 2533-6*

*"Disease arises from, first, dis-ease--as a
normalcy that IS existent and yet becomes
unbalanced. Disease is, or dis-ease is, a
state at variance to the ideal or first cause or
first principle. Then, in its final analysis,
disease might be called sin." 2533-3*

For:

*"...the body-physical becomes that which it
assimilates from material nature. The body-
mental becomes that which it assimilates from
both the physical-mental and the spiritual-
mental. The soul is all of that the entity
is, has been, or may be." 2475-1*

*"...we are physically--that we have digested
for the body.
"We are mentally that which we thought, but it
hasn't added one whit to the physical, has it?
"We are spiritually that we have digested in
our mental beings.
"And if He walks with thee, ye will never be
alone." 2970-1*

Modern medical science is built solely upon the germ theory of disease and of treatment. Ever since the microscope has revealed the presence and seemingly entirely pernicious activity of certain micro-organism in combination with certain diseases, it has been assumed that bacteria are the direct, primary causes of most diseases. Therefore, the slogan now is: "Kill the bacteria (by poisonous antiseptics, serums and antitoxins) and you will cure the disease."

The Edgar Cayce philosophy takes a much different view of the problem. Germs cannot be the cause of disease, because disease germs are also found in the healthiest of bodies. The real cause must, therefore, be something else. Nor is it the waste and morbid matter alone in the system which afford the micro-organisms of disease the opportunity to breed and multiply.

The readings regard micro-organisms as secondary manifestations of illness, and maintain that bacteria and parasites live, thrive, and multiply to the danger point in a weakened, diseased and unbalanced organism only. If it were not so, the human family would become extinct within a few months time.

> "...all illness comes from sin. This everyone must take whether they like it or not; it comes from sin--whether it be of body, of mind or of soul, and these manifest in the earth....
> "And when there are rebellions of body or mind against such, is there any wonder that the atoms of the body cause a rash, or cause indigestion? For, all of these are but the rebellion of truth and light, error and correction in a physical body. For the body is indeed the Temple of the Living God. What have you dragged into this Temple?" 3174-1

The fear instilled by the bacterial theory of disease is frequently more destructive than the micro-organisms themselves. A number of insane patients whose peculiar delusion or monomania was an exaggerated fear of germs, a genine "bacteriophobia."

*"Fear is the root of most of the ills of man-
kind, whether of self, or of what others think
of self, or what self will appear to others.
To overcome fear is to fill the mental, spiritual being with that which wholly casts out
fear; that is as the love that is manifest in
the world through Him who gave Himself the
ransom for many. Such love, such faith, such
understanding, casts out fear. Be not fearful;
for that thou sowest, that thou must reap.
Be more mindful of that sown! 5459-3*

Bacteria are practically omnipresent. We absorb
them in food and drink, we inhale them in the air we
breathe. Our bodies are literally alive with them.
The last stages of the digestive processes depend a
great deal upon the activity of the bacteria in the
intestinal tract.

The primary thing to do, therefore, is not to
try and kill these micro-organisms, but to remove from
the body the cause of sin thereby helping the body to
eliminate the morbid matter and the disease taints in
which they can multiply.

Instead of concentrating energies for killing
germs, whose presence we cannot escape, natural health
applications endeavors to invigorate the system, to
build up blood and lymph on a normal basis, and to
purify the tissues of their morbid encumbrances in
such a way as to establish natural immunity to the
destructive bacterial activities.

Everything that tends to accomplish this without
injuring the system by poisonous drugs or surgical
operations, is acceptable as good, natural healing
treatments.

To adopt the germ-killing process without purifying and invigorating the human organism would be
like trying to keep a house free from fungi and vermin
by sprinkling it daily with carbonic acid and other
germ-killers, instead of keeping it pure and sweet by
flooding it with fresh air and sunshine and applying
freely and vigorously the broom, brush, and plenty
of soap and water. For instead of purifying it, the

antiseptics and germ-killers only add to the filth
of the house.

All bacteriologists are unanimous in declaring
that the various disease germs are found not only in
the bodies of the sick, but also in seemingly healthy
persons.

The inability of bacteria, by themselves, to
create diseases is further confirmed by the well known
fact that certain individuals have a natural immunity
to a specific infection or contagion. All mankind is
more or less affected by hereditary and acquired
disease taints, morbid encumbrances, and drug poisoning, resulting from age-long violation of nature's
laws and from the suppression of acute diseases; but
even under the most universal present conditions of
lowered vitality, morbid hereditary, and physical and
mental degeneration, it is found that under identical
conditions of exposure to drafts or infection, only a
certain percentage of individuals take on or catch a
specific disease.

The fact of natural immunity is constantly confirmed by common experience as well as in the clinics
and laboratories of our medical schools and research
institutes. Of a specific number of mice and rabbits
inoculated with particles of cancer, a very small
percentage of them did not develop the malignant
growth and succumb to its ravages. And so it is with
the human family.

Again:

*"All illness is sin, not necessarily of the
moment, as man counts time, but as a part of
the whole experience. For God has not purposed
or willed that any soul should perish, but
purgeth everyone by illness, by prosperity,
by hardships, by those things needed, in order
to meet self--but in Him, by faith and works,
are ye made every bit whole."* 3395-2

Also:

> *"Sins are of commission and omission. Sins
> of commission were forgiven, while sins of
> omission were called to mind--even by the
> Master."* 281-2

> *"For to know to do good, and do it not, it is
> sin to that soul; and to know the manner, in
> which ye may help others and refrain, it is
> hellish to thine own self, creating conditions
> which must be antagonistic in thine own expe-
> rience with others. It is the law of grace and
> the first law of recompense, the law of love."*
>   5332-1
> *"But remember, as has been given by Him, to
> know to do good and do it not is sin."* 281-30

In this connection it is of interest to learn
that healthy micro-organisms are just as much subject
to dis-eases themselves as they are the by-product of
sin. In their activity as they act as scavengers or
eliminators of morbid matter, they hold in check the
destructive activity of germs and viruses and prevent
their multiplication beyond the danger point. However,
when this expansion becomes extreme, it, nature, as a
natural function, resorts to feverish inflammation as
a warning sign that all is not well within the body.

> *"What has brought distraughtness, distress
> and disease in the earth, or in manifestation,
> is transgression of the Law."* 281-24

On this basis there is then the need to analyze
our own disease situation, for it is but the inevitable
result of violating nature's laws. The first consideration, therefore, is self-examination, in locating
its cause and acting upon it, thus preventing further
expansion of the illness.

However, we must affirm that the dangers from
germs and other infectious diseases lies just as much
or more so in internal filth as in external cleanliness. Cleanliness and asepsis must go hand in hand
with the purification of the inner man in order to

insure "natural immunity," thus creating an atmosphere of harmonious vibratory relationship with life itself.

For:

"There is as much of God in the physical as there is in the spiritual or mental, for it should be one!" 69-21

CHAPTER THREE

THE SYMPHONY OF LIFE

Human life appeared to me as a great orchestra in which we are the players. The great composition to be performed is the Symphony of Life, its infinitude of dissonances and harmonics blending into a single colossal tonal-picture of harmony and grandeur. We players must study the laws of music and the score of the Great Symphony and we must practice diligently and persistently, until we can play our part unerringly in harmony with the concepts of the Great Composer.

At the same time we must learn to keep our own instrument, the body, in the best possible condition; for the greatest artist endowed with a profound knowledge of the laws of music, and possessed of the most perfect technique, cannot produce any musical and harmonious sounds from an instrument with strings too laxed or over tensed, or with the body and mind filled with similarly dissonant tones.

"For remember, music alone may span that space between the finite and the infinite. In the harmony of sound, the harmony of color, even the harmony of motion itself, its beauty is all akin to that expression of the soul-self in the harmony of the mind, if used properly in relationship to body...." 3659-1

"Only music may span that space between the finite and the infinite...music may be the means of arousing and awakening the best of hope, the best of desire, the best in the heart and soul of those who will and do listen. Is not music the universal language, both for those who would give praise and those who are sorry in their hearts and souls? Is it not a means, a manner of universal expression? Thus, may the greater hope come." 2156-1

Therefore, the artist, as each one of us, must learn that the physical instrument, its composition, its construction and its care, are just as much subject to law as the harmonics of the score.

In the final analysis, everything is vibration acting in and on the universal ethers, which are held to be the primordial substance. Possibly even the ethers themselves are but modes of vibrations.

"...But it would also be well to learn the activity of the etheronic and the vibrations of the body, for these are they that produce color, that produce aura, that produce the activities seen AS color." 1436-3

"...that all may vibrate to that thou mayest be able to obtain from the kingdoms that are manifestations of that etheronic energy or that God-energy in the earth...." 440-16

"...etheronic energy is the emanation from the spirit force through the active force of that which makes for matter being held in its positive position, or in its space of activity. Hence thought as a body, whether of an animal or plant, is shown as of plant receiving in its freshness of vigor influences that come from or through the etheronic energy in its activity upon the body, in the expression or upon the plant as in its expression. Hence things that are equal to the same things are equal to each other." 440-13

Accordingly, that which is constructive is in harmonious vibration. That which is destructive is in inharmonious or discordant vibration.

Against this it may be urged that devolution has its harmonics as well as evolution; that every symphony is made of dissonances as well as harmonics. To this I answer: "Unadulterated harmony may, solely for lack of change, become monotonous; but discords alone never create melody, harmony, health or happiness.

The author has come to the belief that, "There
is a principle in nature that impels every entity to
seek vibratory correspondence with another like entity
of opposite polarity." The Cayce readings state that
very same concept in the following:

"...For, as has been in the experience, and as is
partially understood by the entity, everything
in motion, everything that has taken on materiality as to become expressive in any kingdom in
the material world, is by the vibrations that
are the motions--or those positive and negative
influences that make for that differentiation
that man has called matter in its various
stages of evolution into material things."

699-1

Therefore:

"Elements have their attraction and detraction, or those of animosity and those of
gathering together. This we see throughout all
of the kingdoms, as may be termed, whether we
speak of the heavenly hosts or of those of the
stars, or of the planets, or of the various
forces within any or all of same, they have
their attraction or detraction. The attraction
increases that as gives an impulse, that that
becomes the aid, the stimuli, for an impulse
to create. Hence, as may be seen--or may be
brought to man's--that of attraction one for
another gives that stimuli, that impulse to
be the criterion of, or the gratification of,
those influences in the experience of individuals or entities. To smother same oft becomes
deteriorations for each other as may come about
in any form, way or manner. Accidents happen
in creation, as well as in individual's lives!
Peculiar statement here, but--true." 364-6

So as the artist seeks vibratory harmony between
his instrument and the harmonics of the universe of
sound, so the health seeker must ever establish the

vibratory unison between the material elements of his
body and nature's harmonies of health as exist in the
physical universe.

*"What greater joy there be than in the attuning
of the harmonies of nature, the harmonies of
the love of the Father as expressed through
music."* 827-1

*"In the harmony of sound, the harmony of color,
even the harmony of motion itself, its beauty
is all akin to that expression of the soul-
self in the harmony of the mind, if used properly in relationship to body."* 3659-1

Even the atoms and molecules in the wood and
strings of the violin, as well as the sounds produced
from them, are modes of motion or of vibrations. In
order to produce musical and harmonious sounds, the
vibratory conditions of the physical elements of the
violin must be in harmonious vibratory relationship
with nature's harmonies in the universe of sound.

*"Vibrations, to be sure, is an enormous subject.
Though all may not wholly understand what is
accomplished by raising vibrations in self,
or directing vibrations to others; groups or
individuals may aid through the very sincerity
that comes from a closer walk with those Creative Forces. This brings into being the forces
which aid in correlating and coordinating, and
thus meets the combative mental and physical
conditions in the bodies of others."* 281-7

Thus the elements and forces composing the human
body are also vibratory in their nature, the same as
the material elements of the violin. They also must be
kept in a certain well-balanced chemical composition,
mechanical adjustment, and physical refinement, that
they can vibrate in unison with nature's harmonics,
in the physical universe, and thus produce the harmonies of health and strength and beauty within the

body itself.

"The vibrations aid in producing the vibrations necessary, not only for coordination of the glandular system, but for the ability in the nerve itself to be rejuvenated....This works directly upon the glandulary system--the thyroid, the adrenals and the thymus, all the glands of the body; thus enabling them to react as assimilating forces.
"For that is the process or the activity of the glands, to secrete that which enables the body, physically throughout, to reproduce itself." 2475-1

"The activity of the mental or soul forces of the body may control entirely the whole physical (body) through the action of the balance in the sympathetic system, for the sympathetic nerve system is to the soul and spirit forces as the cerebro-spinal is to the physical forces of an entity...." 5717-3

"With, by, and through the mental ability of the entity, or body, to control self, the sympathetic system has often controlled the physical forces of the body, for the body often finds self in this position, if it would allow itself it could fly all to pieces in a moment, but keeps itself much under control of the mental forces, through the sympathetic system--yet at times this reaches the point where almost nerve exhaustion exists. Hence-- rest--quiet--these have often been that factor in the recuperating forces of the body, yet has never corrected that as produces the condition." 943-1

"Might be many things said. The body is excep- tional in the functioning of sympathetic, that especial center of the soul and mental forces."
4359-1

If our own instrument (the body) is put out of
tune, or if we ignorantly or wilfully insist on playing
(activity of the mind) in our own way, regardless of
the score, we naturally produce discords not only for
ourselves, but also create disharmony for our fellow
artists, in the great orchestra of life.

*"Harmony there must be in the experience of
the entity if it will accomplish, if it will
find rest in itself, if it will bring the best
to its fellow men."* 1318-1

Sin, diseases, suffering and evil are nothing but
discords, produced by the ignorance, indifference, or
malice of the players of life. Therefore, we cannot
attribute the discords of life to the Great Composer.
They are of our own making, and will last as long as
we refuse to learn our individual parts and to play
them in tune with the Great Score. For only in this
way can we ever hope to master the art and science
of right living and to enjoy the harmonies of peace,
contentment, and happiness.

*"For, gaining an understanding of the laws as
pertain to right living in all its phases makes
the mind in attune with Creative Forces, which
are of His consciousness."* 262-3

As a result of studying these impressions, experiences, and revelations, as found in the Edgar Cayce
readings, I saw clearly that the conventional methods
of curing individual ailments and social diseases as
applied by our schools of medicine, by our sectarian
religions, social and political lawgivers, and econo-
mists, were only pallative and suppressive, but not
curative; that all these physicians were but tinkering
with effects and symptoms, while entirely ignoring
the underlying causes. I further saw that this palliative or suppressive treatment of disease symptoms,
while their causes are ever allowed to continue must
inevitably result in cumulative effects, aggravating
the diseased condition into a more permanent or chronic

condition. It became evident to me that herein lies the cause of all chronic diseases as found in individual entities, as well as in social and political bodies of all nations of the earth.

"As we find, while there are disturbing conditions and some become very aggravating to the body at times, we find that little, if any, administration here will be of special benefit until there is more peace--or less of consternation within self!...All illness comes from sin. This everyone must take whether he likes it or not; it comes from sin--whether it be of body, of mind, or of the soul..."
3174-1

"For, the beginnings of sin, of course, were in seeking expression of themselves outside of the plan or the way in which God had expressed same. Thus it was the individual, see?"
5749-14

"God, the first cause, in spirit, created in spirit the separate influences or forces that are a portion of, and manifested in the spirit of, God. In that essence, to become materially manifested through the evolution of the spirit of God, sin first began." 262-123

For:

"All forms of sin or lessons may be implied in the word self-ishness." 815-7

"Then we each should know that the sin which lies at our door is ever the sin of selfishness, self-glory, self-honor." 262-114

"Know, self is the only excuse. Self is the only sin; that is selfishness--and all the others are just a modification of that expression of the ego." 1362-1

"For the only sin of man is selfishness!" 987-4

Therefore:

"Be sure your sin will find you out, and that which one counts to self as sin is hiding that which to self's own mind, own intellectuality, is not in accord with physical, moral or spiritual law." 270-15

And:

"It (sin) may be defined in one word disobedience!" 262-125

"That which is brought into materiality is first conceived in spirit. Hence, as we have indicated, all illness is sin, not necessarily of the moment, as man counts time, but as part of the whole experience." 3395-2

However:

"...God hath not purposed or willed that any soul should perish but purgeth everyone by illness, by prosperity, by hardships, by those things needed, in order (for the individual) to meet self. But in Him, by faith and works, are ye made every whit whole." 3395-2

"Is thy hell one that is filled with fire or brimstone? But know, each and every soul is tried so as by fire, purified, purged; for He, though He were the Son, learned obedience through the things which He suffered. Ye also are known even as ye do, and have done." 281-16

"Remember, for every individual physical body what might be sometimes called symptoms are ever present. But the breaking of cells, injury to some portions of the body, these are usually the sources and the activities that bring about such. The body here is growing more healthy and less susceptible to such disturbances." 533-18

CHAPTER FOUR

HARMONICS OF THE
PHYSICAL, MENTAL, SPIRITUAL

In all the definitions of the constructive and destructive principles in nature, the Cayce readings emphasize the fact that these two same forces are at work in all of the kingdoms of life, from the lowest to the highest. It follows then, that they must be active also in the human body, from its smallest cellular movement to its highest creative activity.

> "In the beginning there was the force of attraction and the force that repelled. Hence, in man's consciousness he became aware of what is known as the atomic or cellular form of movement about which there becomes nebulous activity. And this is the lowest form (as man would designate) that's in active forces in his experience. Yet this very movement that separates the forces in atomic influence is the first cause, or the manifestation of that called God in the material plane.
> "Then, as it gathers of positive and negative forces in their activity, whether it be of one element or realm or another, it becomes magnified in its force or sources through the universe." 262-52

> "To be sure, the entity recognizes that there are the two great forces manifested in the experience of individuals, just as indicated first by the lawgiver and then by the Master Himself: 'There is today set before thee good and evil, life and death.' There are the manifestations of each of these influences, as expressed in Him who is the life and the light of the world, who gave that these were the works whereby there was manifested unto the

world the power of the All Creative Force."
967-3

"As has been given by Him, the power as attained by the study that has been shown in the first portions is to be applied, or may be applied unworthily--as is shown by the beast with two ways, two horns. Then here, how hath it been given? One Lord, one faith, one God, one baptism, one way! Yet in the experience as ye watch about you there are constantly shown the influences by the very forces of the beast with the double-mindedness, as showing wonders in the earth yet they must come even as He hath given, 'Though ye may have done this or that, though ye may have healed the sick, though ye may have cast out demons in my name, I know ye not; for ye have followed rather as the beast of self-aggrandizement, self-indulgence, self-glorification, even as the beast shown here." 281-34

The constructive and destructive principles may seem obvious and self-evident, nevertheless it needs to be emphasized, because there seems to be much confusion of thought on this simple proposition, even among those who should know better.

Many students of the higher philosophy, of new thought, occultism and meta-physics, have centered all their attention and their efforts so thoroughly upon the higher planes that they overlook the existence of and the necessity for compliance with the natural laws of the physical plane. They seem to assume that so long as they understand and comply with the laws on the higher planes, affairs on the lower plane will take care of themselves. They are like the artist who understands all about the laws of music and commands a perfect technique, and therefore, does not think it necessary or worth while to keep his instrument in perfect condition or attunement.

"So seldom is it considered by all, that spirituality, mentality and the physical

*being are all one; yet may indeed separate
and function one without the other--and one at
the expense of the other. Make them cooperative, make them one in their purpose--and we
will have a greater activity."* 307-10

*"There are three influences then in the system
or in the body; the body-mental, the body-
physical, the body-spiritual. They are one;
yet they each in their own sphere...of weaknesses, must function and rely upon those
activities to which the body-mental, the body-
physical activities add to the foods--not only
bodily foods but the thinking foods, for the
resuscitation and revivification for the activities."* 1158-3

Therefore:

*"Each soul, individual or entity, finds these
facts existent:*
*"There is the body-physical--with all of its
attributes for the functioning of the body in
a three-dimensional or a manifested earth
plane.*
*"Also there is the body-mental--which is that
directing influence of the physical, the mental
and the spiritual emotions and manifestations
of the body; or the way, the manner...as to
things, conditions and circumstances...*
*"Then there is the body-spiritual, or the
soul-body.. that eternal consciousness in which
the individual entity in patience becomes
aware of its relationship to the mental and
the physical being.*
*"All of these are one--in an entity; just as
is considered, realized or considered that
the body, mind and soul are one--that God,
the Son, and the Holy Spirit are one."* 2475-1

After all, physical health is the best possible
basis for the attainment of mental, moral and spiritual

health. All building begins with the foundation. We do not first suspend the steeple in the air and then build the church under it. So also, does building the temple of human character begin by laying down the foundation of physical health.

Many of us have known people who have attained high intellectual, moral, and spiritual development, and then suffered utterly becoming as shipwrecks, physically, mentally and in every other way, because they ignorantly had violated the laws of their own physical nature.

There are others who believe that the possession of occult knowledge and the achievement of mastership, confers absolute control over nature's forces and its phenomena on the physical plane. These people believe a man is not a master if he does not heal all manner of disease and create various miracles. Now if such things were possible, they would be able to overthrow the laws of cause and effect, of karma, and of compensation. They would be able to abolish and nullify the basic structural principles of morality and its constructive influences.

If it is possible in one case to heal disease and to overcome death through the fiat of the will of a master, then it must be possible in all cases. If so, then we can ignore the existence of nature's laws, indulge our appetites and our passions to the fullest extent, and when the obvious results of our transgressions overtake us, we can go to one of the many healers, or masters, and have all of our diseases "instantly and painlessly" removed, like having a bad tooth extracted by a dentist.

But:

"...first of all, let the body know this:
"Not palliatives but healing that is sincere
--of whatever nature, whether spiritual,
magnetic, mechanical, even drugs, electrical,
heat, or whatever application--to be of real
aid for the body--must bear the imprint or
stamp of the universal or divine. No matter

*in what sphere or plane a soul may find itself;
this law is ever the same!
"Construction and constructive influences can
only emanate from good. Good can only emanate
from God.
"Hence, that which may be healing in every
nature--any nature--can only come from one
source.Palliatives may be injected for a time;
but half a truth is worse than a whole lie,
for it decimateth even the soul!" 366-1*

*"Healing for the physical body, then, must be
first the correct choice of the spiritual
import held as the ideal of the individual.
For it is returning, of course, to the First
Cause--First Principles." 2528-2*

I say this with all due reverence for, and faith
in, the efficacy of true prayer, with full knowledge
of the healing power of therapeutic faith, that God,
I do not believe, or that nature, a master, or meta-
physical formula, can or will ever make good, in a
miraculous way, for the inevitable results of our
transgressions of the natural laws governing our being
without its due compensation.

If such miraculous healings were at all possible
on demand, and of common occurrence, what occassion
would there be for the exercise of Reason, Will and
Self-control? What would become of the spiritual basis
of sincere morality and its constructive applications.

All this leads us to the following conclusions:

If there is in operation a constructive principle
of nature on the ethical, moral, mental and spiritual
planes of being, with which we must align ourselves,
and to which we must conform our conscious and voluntary activities in order to achieve self-completion,
self-contentment, individual completion and true happiness. Then this constructive principle must be in
operation also in our physical bodies, and in their
co-related physical, mental and spiritual activities.
If the constructive principle is active in the physical
as well as in the moral, mental and spiritual realms,

then the established harmonic relationship of the physical to the constructive law of its being must constitute the morality of the physical, and from this it follows then that the achievement of health on the physical plane is as much under our conscious and voluntary control as the working out of our individual salvation or karma on the higher planes of life.

To recapitulate-- First: Our well-being on all planes and in all relationships of life depends upon the existence, recognition and practical application of the same great principle and fundamental laws of nature as found throughout the universe.

"For all laws (loves) that are applicable in a material world must find their inception, their beginning, in the source of that beginnings of activity in a given sphere.
"The forces of spirit activity, then, become all those that are recognized as the elemental laws, or what?
"First, self-perpetuation or preservation; perpetuation through second law of its creation, through its elements that partake of the life spirit that creates or forms the body itself. Hence we have the first three laws in the activity of spirit in matter in the earth!
"Preservation of self; preservation in perpetuation of self, by impregnation of matter to become a reproduction of itself; and-- like begets like!" 3744-1

"There are laws, then, as govern the physical, the mental, the spiritual body, and the attributes of each of these. The abuse of a physical law brings dis-ease and then disturbance to the physical organism, through which mental and spiritual portions of the body operate."
1947-3

Second: Physical health, as well as moral and mental health, is of our own making. We are personnaly responsible, not only for our own physical and mental health, but we are also morally responsible for the

hereditary tendencies of our offsprings toward health
or disease.

*"That the sins of the fathers are visited
unto the children of the third and fourth
generation, even to the tenth. This is not
saying that the results are seen only in the
bodily functions of the descendants, as is
ordinarily implied; but that the essence of the
message is given to the individual respecting
the activity of which he may or must eventually
be well aware in his own being. That is, what
effects does it have upon you to even get mad,
to laugh, to cry, to be sorrowful? All of
these activities affect not only yourself,
your relationships to your fellow man, but
your next experience in the earth!"* 281-38

*"To be sure, those things which have to do
with body-mind activities of an entity are the
physical results of conditions which existed
in the experience of the parent of the entity
--as well as in the experience of their parents.
For it is a fact that there are as circumstances and conditions which arise in the
genealogical reactions which go back--as
indicated in the Law--'unto the third and
fourth generations.'*
*"These, then, are tendencies and inclinations
which may arise in bodies, provided such bodies
are not aware of them and do not take measures
to correct such weaknesses or tendencies,
found to be a part of the entity's physical
experience."* 2533-4

*"The weaknesses that exist in this particular
body are a projection of those conditions which
existed in the great-grandfather of the entity,
in an experience in the earth; and has to do
with those elements bearing upon the hormones
of the blood force itself...*
"To eradicate, to eliminate such from the

*body is to interpret that which was given in
the beginning: 'Be ye fruitful, multiply, but
subdue' the tendencies and the inclinations
of the 'earth.' For the spiritual and mental
forces manifest in the earth, they partake of
the earth. And the earth is earthy, in that
it changes. It is in constant change." 2533-4*

*"...the entity, were it able--will it arouse
within self that that will be able to subdue
the passions of those influences which have
become inherent from the indiscretions of the
youth of the parents of the entity--there
will be brought the full knowledge and understanding that the truth in Him makes one free
indeed, and though the law says that 'I will
visit the afflictions of the fathers upon the
children to the third and fourth generation,'
so also is that healing as comes through the
gift of the Son into the world, that 'Though
thy sins be as scarlet they shall be white
like wool.'" 543-1*

Third: The attainment of physical health through
compliance with nature's laws is just as much a part
of the Great Work as our ethical, moral and psychical
development for becoming a good citizen.

*"Then, as the entity in this material plane
has found, it is necessary physically to
conform to certain moral and penal laws of
society, of the state, of the nation, even to
be termed a good citizen. Thus if there is
to be preparation for the entity as the soul-
entity, as a citizen of the heavenly kingdom,
isn't it just as necessary that there be the
conforming to the laws pertaining to that
spiritual kingdom of which this entity is a
part?" 3590-2*

Fourth: Ignorance of the laws is not a presump-
tion for their non-activity or existence.

*"Individuals we find carry out certain elements
and laws, and gradually man becomes capable
of applying and using these in the everyday
life of man. This, whether applied in medical
science, in anatomical science, in mechanical
science or what not, is merely the development,
or the application as man applies to Universal
laws as are ever, and have ever been, existent
in the Universe."* 900-70

Fifth: All laws are interrelated one with another.

*"There are divine or universal laws, as there
are nature's laws--as well as man's laws.
For one is the attempt to understand the other,
or one is the searching for the other."* 2615-1

*"Causes and effects are evident in a material
world. While one follows the other, they are
as interlocking as day and night."* 343-2

Sixth: The immutable law of cause and effect:

*"The law of cause and effect is immutable, by
choice in individual experience. Or choice is
the factor that alters or changes the effect
produced by that which is the builder for every
experience of associations of man, in even
material experience. Hence as thought, and
purpose, and aim, and desire, are set in motion
by minds, their effect is as a condition that
IS. For its end, then, has been set in that
He, the Giver of the heavens and the earth
and those things therein, has set the end
thereof."* 262-83

*"The immutable law of cause and effect is, as
evidenced in the world today, in the material,
the mental and the spiritual world, but He--
in overcoming the world, the law--became the
Law. The law then, becomes as the schoolmaster,
or the school of training--and we who have*

*named the Name, then, are no longer under the
law as law, but under mercy as in Him; for in
Him--and with the desires--may there be made
the coordination of all things." 262-36*

Seven: The law of karma. *"That which is cosmic,
or destiny, or karma..." 276-7*

*"As has been given, it will be long, it will
be tedious; but, as has been given, this is
a duty from those to whom the body has come.
If it is held as that which must be met, that
they and the body itself may enjoy in material
associations the pleasures of the activity of
the spiritual forces well.
"The same with individuals where there is in
their experience crosses to bear, hardships
or surroundings that to them are overpowering,
overwhelming, by slights, slurs, and fancies
of the inactivity of a coordinating force.
If these are held continually as crosses, or
as things to be overcome, then they will remain
as crosses. But if they are to be met with
the spirit of truth and right in their own
selves, they should create joy; for that is
what will be built.
"For, the Father of light has never failed man
that has cried in earnestness unto Him. It is
when individuals have desired their own way
that the souls have suffered in the sons of
men." 552-2*

Eight: The law of grace is the law of mercy and
nullifies all of the others.

*"Then as the entity sets itself to do or to
accomplish that which is of creative influence
or force, it comes under the interpretation of
the law between karma and grace. No longer is
the entity under the law of cause and effect,
or karma, but rather in grace it may go on to
the higher calling in Him." 2800-2*

Therefore:

"*For what one sows that must one reap. This is unchangeable law. Know that this law may be turned into law of grace and mercy by the individual, through living and acting in their lives in relationships to others.*" 5233-1

"*...meeting those things which have been called karmic, yet remembering that under the law of grace this may not be other than an urge, and that making the will of self one with the Way may prevent, may overcome, may take the choice that makes for life, love, joy, happiness-- rather than the law that makes, causes the meeting of everything the hard way.*
"*For the self is constantly meeting self.*"
                                                1771-2

However:

"*Though one may have the gift of graces in Hope, in Charity, in Faith, and has not the law of Love in their heart, soul, mind, and though they give their body to give itself for manifesting even these graces, and has not love--they are nothing.*" 3744-4

Let us analyze, therefore, what has been brought forth above in relationship to our own individual-istic experiences.

"*In analyzing the disturbances which exists here, it would be well for the body to analyze much of its attitude that has been overcome-- in a measure...While the body has been and is a very good anatomist; it finds (that) impulses received through the mind and through the radiation of vibration on environment have often had much to do with the manner in which an organ, a nerve, a gland will respond to stimulations made from the administration of many characters of combinations of drugs or*

even mechanical applications. They do not respond the same under some conditions as under some others. Why?
"There is a body, there is a mind, there is soul. They each have their attributes, they each have their limitations. The soul, in a material world, is controlled by mind and body.
"Then these all should be taken into consideration. Then the body will interpret, will see how that resentments that have been a part of the experience of the entity through periods of its development have had their influence. Yes, they were brought from other experiences also. Much has been done about it, and thus much may be done about these conditions--if there will be the correct attitude of the body in making application of certain elements as to coordinate with the disturbance existent in the body."
3559-1
"This may be answered, even as was that 'Who sinned, this man or his parents?' That the works of God might be manifest before you! When there are karmic conditions in the experience of an individual, that as designates those that have the Christ-like spirit is not only in praying for them, holding meditation for them, but aiding, helping in every manner that the works of God may be manifest in their lives, and every meditation or prayer: 'Thy will, O God, be done in that body as Thou seest best.' 'Would that this cup might pass from me, not my will but Thine be done.'" 281-4

And:

"...who bringeth this or that (illness or health) to pass in thy experience in order that, through thy experience ye may learn the more of the law of the Lord, learn that it is perfect?" 2828-4

Thus:

*"Remember, the sources (of this body'y con-
dition), as we have indicated are the meeting
of one's own self! Thus they are karmic.
"These can be met most in Him who, taking away
the law of cause and effect by fulfilling the
law, establishes the law of grace. Thus the
need is for the entity to lean upon the arm of
Him who is the law, and the truth and the
light."* 2828-4

But:

*"One may preserve youth, even as is desired,
will they pay the price as is necessary; but
one adding this, that, or the other to the
system to become congenial with that known
from within self is an abnormality to itself,
must pay its price."* 900-465

*"For here we have an individual entity meeting
its own self--the conditions in regards to
the movements of the body, the locomotories,
the nerve ends, the muscular forces. What ye
demanded of others (in another experience) ye
must pay yourself! Every soul should remember
not to demand of others more than ye are
willing to give, for ye will pay and as most,
through thy gills."* 3845-1

So:

*"Remember, the things you applied once--now
you are meeting them! Live with this in mind
(and every soul may take heed): YOU SHALL PAY
EVERY WHIT THAT YOU BREAK OF THE LAW OF THE
LORD. For the Law of the Lord is perfect, it
converteth the soul."* 3559-1

CHAPTER FIVE

THE UNITY AND CONTINUITY OF THE LAW

That which we call God, Nature, the Creator, or
the Creative Force, is the great central cause of all
things. And the vibratory activities produced by or
proceeding from this central or primary cause, or First
Cause, may continue through all spheres of life in
like manner, as the light waves of the sun, moon, and
fixed stars penetrate through the intervening sphere
of light of our own planet earth. Therefore, all powers,
forces, laws and principles which manifest on our
plane, proceed and continue from the innermost Divine
to the most external plane in physical nature. This
explains the unity and continuity, stability and
creativity, correspondingly existing on all planes of
being, of that called "Natural Law." In other words,
"Natural Law" is the established harmonic relationship
of effects and phenomena to their causes, and for all
particular causes to the one great primary cause or
the First Cause of all things.

And Cayce states:

"What is the First Cause?
"That which has brought, is bringing, all life
into being; or animation, or force, or power,
or movement, or consciousness, as to either
the material plane, the mental plane, the
spiritual plane. Hence it is the force that
is called Lord, God, Jehovah, Yah, Ohum, (ohm),
Abba and the like." 254-67

"What then was--or is--the First Cause? For
if there be law pertaining to the First Cause
it must be an unchangeable law, and is--IS as
I AM that I AM! For this is the basis from
which one would reason.

49

*"The first cause was, that the created would
be the companion for the Creator, that it,
the creature, would show itself to be not only
worthy of, but companionable to, the Creator.
"Hence every form of life that man sees in a
material world is an essence or manifestation
of the Creator; not the Creator, but a manifestation of a first cause, and in its own
sphere, its own consciousness of its activity
in that plane or sphere." 5753-1*

These truths became revealed to me, in their
fullest significance and universal application, when
I became acquainted with the readings of Edgar Cayce.
I then perceived the identity and perfect correspondence of the laws and principles which underlie the
"Great Work," the "Bible," on the spiritual, mental,
ethical, moral and psychical planes, and the result-
ant natural healing philosophy on the physical plane.
The central truth in the philosophy of the Cayce
readings is, that universal laws are active throughout
nature as they are within the nature of man himself.
There are, therefore, in nature, two great fundamental
principles of opposite tendencies namely, a constructive and destructive principle, and that all activities
in nature and in human nature align themselves with,
and come under the action of one of those controlling
principles.

The readings speak of nature as follows:

*"Nature is that from which man may take his
lesson to learn of the Creative Forces or God."
5214-1
"...there is within the grasp of man all that
in nature that is the counterpart of that in
the mental and spiritual realms and an antidote
for every poison, for every ill in the individual experience, if there will but be applied
nature, natural sources." 2396-2*

"...for he that is close to nature, he that

*is close to the manifesting of life in its
primitive form...keeps close to that way
wherein a knowledge of the Creative Forces may
be made manifest in self." 3000-2*

Therefore:

*"...man in his nature--physical, mental and
spiritual--is a replica, is a part of the whole
universe reaction in materiality." 3492-1*

In other terms, man has a spiritual individuality,
a mental individuality as well as a physical individuality. Moreover, these are all subject to the very
general principles of integration and disintegration,
construction and destruction as is found throughout
the universe itself.

The mental individuality of a highly intelligent
man or woman is as truly a result of growth as are
his physical and spiritual organisms. In other words,
it is the result of unfoldment, integration and construction. The principle back of it is known as the
"Constructive Principle" of nature at work influenc-
ing the individual life.

*"Then, as the mind is the builder, keep the
mind upon constructive influences; knowing
that the Creative Force or God is mindful of
thee--as thou art a part of that universal
consciousness." 2386-1*

*"As you then sow constructive influences into
the lives and experiences of others, you make
such growth in your relationships to the
WHOLE." 1463-1*

*"When the mental self is loosed in the quietness
of those periods when it would take cognizance
of the influences about self, we find the
mental as a vapor, as a gas, (not that it is
either, but as comparison) is loosened by the
opening of the self through those centers of*

*the body that arouses the awareness of the
mental to the indwelling of the spiritual
self that is a portion of and encased within
self. And it, the energy, to the temple of the
motivative forces of the physical body." 826-11*

But we also all know that there is a principle
in nature which when set in motion upon the physical
plane, disintegrates our physical bodies, tears them
down, destroys their individualities and resolves them
back into the elements from which they were built up.
We also know that there is a principle or process,
which, when it becomes dominant in human life, tears
down or destroys the individuality of human intelligence. With the same unerring certainty we know that
there is in nature that which, when it becomes a
dominant factor in human nature, tears down, dissi-
pates, or destroys the most beautiful individualities
of the highest moral character.

*"When the mental is attuned to those that
become of a self-exaltation, of self-aggrandizement of those forces as build for material,
or those that build for the gratification of
selfish--or of self's desire, irrespective
of the other--these must become destructive
in their final analysis..." 1735-2*

*"That which is of a selfish or a self-indulgent
nature, or for self-aggrandizement, is destructive; and is naturally then destructive in
the experience of an entity." 1431-1*

*"The destructive energies, then, are in the
greater portion active through the vegetative
and sympathetic nerve systems--as related to
either a portion of the lower portion of the
stomach proper where assimilation first begins
to take place, or through the organs of distribution of blood supply so assimilated."*
5497-1

That which disintegrates, tears down, or destroys

any of nature's constructive influences in individualities, whether they be spiritual, mental, emotional
or physical has been designated as the "Destructive
Principle" of nature acting within individuals.

Therefore:

*"The attitude of mind makes for that which
gives the birth, or the rising up of peace,
harmony, understanding, or it is as the children of the mind--that which brings contend-
ing forces that may be warred against; for as
all must find, 'When I would do right the
spirit of unrest is ever present.' As day by
day this is put out of the mind, and more and
more the mind of harmony, peace, understanding
--not a latent kind, but an active force--so
does this become the manner in which self is
giving expression of that being sought."*

262-3

The different attitudes of mind, whether in its
departments of thought or feeling, are well known to
exert a powerful influence upon the physiological
manifestations; but unfortunately the considerations
of these relations has been too generally left to a
class of writers whose aim is to astonish and amuse
rather than to effect any practical good for their so
called disquisitions.

We hear it constantly asserted by invalids, that
some peculiar mental trouble, disappointment, or excitement of feeling was the original cause of their
ill health. But how very few think of looking for
relief, or are led to look for it, in a restoration
of order and harmony to the disturbed mind. How few
seem to know that the forces that exercise such potent
control over the organism for the production of disease,
may be made equally available for the restoration of
health. The ordinary practice of medicine inculcates
the notion that the business of the physicians is
simply to endeavor to supply and regulate certain
material conditions, by means of pill and powder, and
that when that is accomplished, all has been done

that lie within the limits of human ability.

The truth is, the influence of the mind over the body is equally great in health and in disease. No thoughful observer can doubt this. We have seen the voluntary muscular action giving language to those ideas, and that no part of the framework of the body is ever exempt from the duties of aiding in the performance of this interesting and wonderful function. All these external manifestations depend upon certain changes effected among the invisible elements of matter.

> *"Remember, the mental attitudes will have much to do with whether you will grow a straight toenail or keep your eyes straight, or keep your voice when you are upset. For these work with the glands of the sensory system.*
> *"...remember that the attitude of mind has much to do with the conditions of the body-- this body particularly." 2376-1*

Now the extraordinary states into which this system may be thrown into, soon subsides and are then directly succeeded by the ordinary or normal states, and whether the impressions thus made are wholesome or unwholesome, the effects are not necessarily permanent. But if these destructive conditions are to be continued for any considerable length of time, the consequence will be serious, and may even be fatal. The continued indulgence of malicious feelings by a person, for example, will surely so modify all the internal invisible functional acts of the system as to check and overcome finally its vital power; and thus any latent tendencies to chronic disease that may belong to the person will certainly be quickened into active life.

> *"For as has been indicated in some manners, some activities, there is an activity within the system produced by anger, fear, mirth, joy, or any of those active forces, that produces through the glandular secretion those activities that flow into the whole of the*

system. Such an activity then is of this endocrine system, and only has been observed in very remote manners, or just here and there. Only the more recently has this activity received that consideration from the specialist in ANY activity in the relationships to the human body." 281-38

"To be sure, attitudes often influence physical conditions of the body, No one can hate his neighbor and not have stomach or liver trouble. No one can be jealous or allow the anger from it, without having upset digestion or heart disorder." 4021-1

Therefore, a grave difficulty to be encountered in overcoming states of chronic disease by ordinary medical means is now seen. Diseases are perpetuated, if not produced, by destructive causes over which mere chemical influences can not be presumed to so exercise any positive control over such negative attitudes. This fact may be, often is, tacitly acknowledged by the physician, but he declines to investigate its relationships so as to be able to turn them to useful accounts. He is unwilling to acknowledge in practice, although he may admit confidentially, that headaches, nervousness, heart disease, or the dyspeptic qualms which he is called upon to remedy, are only but the indications of some peculiar morbid state of mind. Or perhaps it is but the emotional nature of the sufferer, which it becomes him to meet directly, rather than to torment his patient with an eternal round of palliatives.

In these cases, every medical prescription must be totally irrelevant (although written in the best Latin) unless it recognizes the operation of causes existing in a sphere quite beyond the reach of the most potent drug. What fatal mistakes may not result when stimuli are substituted for encouragement, and physics for rational ideas; when the invalid is advised to try the resources of an inexhaustible pharmacy, instead of bringing common sense to a controlling sway

in the organism! Neither physician nor patient can
afford any longer to devote his attention exclusively
to the superficial and deceptive signs of disease, nor
to ignore the fact, that the body is but the incarnate
expression of the interior, invisible, imperishable
spirit, which exist in and is part of man himself.

*"More often we think of spirit as just a name,
rather than experiencing it. Yet we use it,
we manifest it, we are a part of it. Taking
THOUGHT doesn't change anything! It is the
application of the thought taken that makes
the change within ourselves!" 262-119*

*"...the Spirit is of the Creator, and thy
body is the temple of that Spirit manifested
in the earth to defend or to use in thine
own ego, or thine own self-indulgence, or to
thine own glory, OR unto the glory of Him who
gave thee life and immortality--if ye preserve
that life, that Spirit in Him." 2448-2*

We can never get rid of the sequences of this
important fact, that in the human organism spirit
governs matter, by brutishly ignoring it; nor can we
innocently treat it as an unimportant matter. Science,
like true religion, is learning every day to live
more and more by faith and less by sight.

The jests that used to be hurled at the defense-
less head of the practioner who dared to suggest that
the thoughts and feelings and mental habits of the
invalid might need rectifying as well as his bile and
blood, are fast losing their point. We are beginning
to suspect that perhaps, after all, a disease may not
be the less a disease because its source happens to
lie in an unruly imagination, or in excessive negative
activity, or a wrong mode of thought. And gradually--
very slowly, to be sure--yet really, we think people
are waking up to the conviction that these intangible
causes are not irremediable. They are now beginning to
see and understand that by this close union and co-
operation of the material and the immaterial natures,

remedial agents may possibly find access to either or both through avenues that otherwise could have no existence. We have faith to believe that the time is near at hand when the mental aspects and its relationships to disease will then receive an amount of such attention as to be equal to that which has always been given to the beat of the pulse and condition of the tongue, the temperature of the skin and the color and consistence of the excretions of the body.

Blessed will be the day when science shall purge her soul of the dishonor of leaving this interesting and vital subject to ignorance and charlatanry. But even the devil should have his due. As much as we all detest quackery, it can not be denied that many quacks meet with a success in the treatment of some diseases that would be very puzzling if we could not refer it in great measure to the mental control they contrive to exert over their patients. In this respect, in its practice, the pretender has a positive and oftentimes an immense advantage over the real man of science. He stimulates his patient's imagination, awakens his hope, gains his confidence, whereby the perturbed mind is restored to a condition of tranquility, and thus a state of the system is induced most conducive to that spontaneous restoration of its harmony and power which is often mistaken for the effect of medication.

A wholesome co-operation of the mental, emotional, and material forces of the invalid is, indeed, that grand desideratum, and if the charlatan can secure it, he is certainly entitled to the credit of doing what his betters have so often and so lamentably failed in their efforts to accomplish.

Every one knows what benefit is frequently derived from a simple change of doctors; this benefit is thus generally much greater than the difference that the courses of treatment will account for. We all know how salutary are the influences of a cheerful society, change of scenery, and exciting incidents, in some conditions of the system. It is very strange that the abundant experiences of men in this direction should not have long ago convinced them of the existence of laws and principals so important and so fundamental.

No attempt is made herein at giving any specific directions in regard to the best manner of bringing the principles and laws of mental and physical health to bear upon particular cases. We can only direct en passant the attention of individuals, invalids and physicians, to this important subject. No extensive practical advantage, however, will be reaped until these principles and laws are taught in our schools and incorporated into our medical science.

The philosophy and teachings of the Edgar Cayce readings, as far as is laid down in the transcript records, deal mainly with the application of these immutable laws and principles to our ethical, moral, spiritual and psychical development. It remained, however, for the followers of the Cayce philosophy to demonstrate that the same laws and principles which form the exact and mathematical basis for ethics, morality and positive mentality, controls with equal force and precision the processes of health, disease and cure within the physical body and its correlated physical, mental and emotional activities. The key here, that opens the door, is application.

> *"Remember, one must be open-minded, open-hearted. Forgive and forget. Remember, too, that by applying truths known, you come to know greater truths. Only by application--even if by rule or rote--you may find the true meaning of laws. And this is true of laws pertaining to the mind, or the physical body, or the spiritual body." 967-1*

> *"And the application of that received there, then, in thy physical consciousness, physical mind--applied in thy relationships to those ye meet day by day--causes the growth to come."*
> *826-11*

The readings state that only in the application does the understanding comes, for it is the law.

> *"In the application of that as has been gained comes the understanding." 262-18*

"For it is in the application, not the knowledge, that the truth becomes a part of thee."
                                        826-11

Therefore:

"In application the meaning of a theory is understood. As has been given, to know and not to do is sin. To know, and to apply that which is known, gives growth in understanding."
                                        900-429

However:

"When there is the application rather for self-indulgence, self-aggrandizement, or only for material gains, then it eventually brings distortion, disturbance and distress—even into the material and the mental and the spiritual aspects of an entity." 1862-1

And:

"One grows in grace, in knowledge and in understanding by perfecting the application of truths within the self. For only application brings spiritual and mental growth, to and through action." 2756-1

"As given, each in their own way and manner may aid, or hinder, according to the application of their own abilities, own talent, own understanding." 262-7

"Apply ye that ye know, for in the application comes understanding. For, as the Master gave, 'Ye are Gods.' if ye will use His force of desire and will in His kingdom, but NOT thine own." 262-64

"...the material effects then may be the result of the spiritual application. And not the material the goal, but as the result of soul development." 1219-1

"In application, this as is seen comes from and thru that which finding a truth of any character, information of any nature as is related and is relating to the endeavor of the one making such an application, and is then of the personal, rather than of the general or universal nature, and in application one begins to understand, for as has been given, the growth is from within, for first appears the blade, then the flower, and then the whole fruit, ripe and ready to be applied to the usages of others. Do not attempt to walk before crawling. Do not run before one is able to walk. Feed not children upon meats, and keep thine own heart pure." 900-323

A man may bestow the greatest care upon what he eats and drinks; and regulate ever so faithfully his periods of exercise and of repose; and learn by heart whole treatises on the art of living long; profoundly reflect on the relationship of his feelings, his will and thoughts to his general well-being. But more than this is demanded of him. He must learn to govern, as well as to know himself. Does the reader say, "Oh, I am incapable of such efforts as are necessary for this." I answer: Your duty in the premises is demonstrable, God who succors the raven so tenderly, is not a hard Master. "You can do what you should do."

CHAPTER SIX

HEALING: AN EXACT SCIENCE

One of the reasons why natural healing is not more popular with the medical profession and the public is that it is too simple. The average mind is much more impressed by the involved and the mysterious than by the simple and common-sense approach.

However, it remains a fact that at times medical science reduces complexity and confusion to simplicity and clearness. Its science becomes exact science only when the underlying laws which co-relate and unify its scattered facts and theories have been discovered. The wonderful structures of modern astronomy and chemistry and physics have been elaborated from a few basic laws and principles of nature, such as the laws of gravitation, the laws of polarity and chemical affinity.

What the discovery of these natural laws has done for astronomy and chemistry, the fundamental laws and principles of natural healing philosophy will similarly do for medical science. They will reduce chaos and confusion to simplicity, and obscurity to clarity, and will thereby change what was pure empiricism to an exact healing science.

"Let's analyze healing for the moment, to those that must consciously...see and reason, see a material demonstration, occasionally at least! Each atomic force of a physical body is made up of its units of positive and negative forces, that brings it into a material plane. These are of the ether, or atomic forces, being electrical in nature as they enter into a material basis, or become matter in its ability to take on or throw off. So, as a group may raise the atomic vibrations that make for those positive forces as bring divine forces in action into a material plane, those that

61

are destructive are broken down by the raising
of that vibration! That's material, see? This
is done through Creative Forces, which are God
in manifestation! Hence, as self brings those
little things necessary, as each is found to
be necessary, for position, posture, time,
period, place, name, understanding, study
each, and assist each in their respective
sphere. So does the entity become the healer.

                                        281-3

"As we have indicated, the body-physical is an
atomic structure subject to the laws of its
environment, its hereditary, its soul development. The activity of healing, then, is to
create or make a balance in the necessary units
of the influence or force...

"It is seen that each atom, each corpuscle, has
within same the whole form of the universe...

"As for the physical body, this is made up of
the elements of the various natures that keep
same in its motion necessary for sustaining
its equilibrium; as begun from its (the individual body's) first cause.

"If in the atomic forces there becomes an overbalancing, an injury, a happening, an accident,
there are certain atomic forces destroyed or
others increased; that to the physical body
become either such as to add to or take from
the elan vital that makes for the motivative
forces through that particular...activity.

"Then, in meeting these it becomes necessary
for the creating of that influence within each
individual body to bring a balance necessary
for its continued activity about each of the
atomic centers its own rotary or creative force,
...for the ability of resuscitating, revivi-
fying, such influence or force in the body."

                                        281-24

"...all healing of every nature is the changing
of the vibrations from within--the attuning of
the divine within the living tissue of a body
to Creative Energies. Whether it is accom-

*plished by the use of drugs, the knife or
what not, it is the attuning of the atomic
structure of the living cellular force to its
spiritual heritage." 1967-1*

*"For, all healing comes from the one source.
And whether there is the application of
foods, exercise, medicine, or even the knife
--it is to bring the consciousness of the
forces within the body that aid in reproducing
themselves--the awareness of Creative or God
Forces." 2696-1*

The most important of the natural remedies can
be had free of any cost and are found in every earthly
home. They are: Fresh Air (AIR); Fasting (EARTH); Water
(WATER); and Emotions (FIRE). In the heavenly home
they are Right Attitude (BODY), Prayer (MIND) and
Meditation (SPIRIT). In these we find the seven aspects
of nature at work in the nature of man manifesting
through the seven glandular centers of the endocrine
system of the body.

I am fully aware and convinced that these remedies
offered freely by mother nature are sufficient and,
if rightly applied, can cure any disease arising within
the organism of man. If circumstances permit however,
we may advantageously add: Corrective Manipulation,
such as massage, osteopathic and chiropractic treatments, herb and homeopathic remedies.

These truths may be expressed in another way. The
victory of these healing forces in acute diseases
depends upon an abundant supply of electro-magnetic
energies. The positive mental attitude of faith and
equanimity creates positive vital energies in the body
thus infusing the battling phagocytes with increased
vigor and favoring the secretion of antitoxins and
anti-bodies, while the negative, fearful and worrying
attitude of mind, creates in the system the negative
condition of weakness, lowered resistance, which can
sometimes even cause actual paralysis.

"The manner of overcoming such, as has been

intimated, may best be accomplished by the laying on of hands. This enables the entity being aided to have something to hold on to --something that is as concrete as the illness with which he is battling. Then by cooperative and concerted action of the group--and by the laying on of hands, there will come--we find --a complete cure." 281-5

"As we have indicated, use more of the magnetic forces in the application of healing influence to others; not discounting that already applied but the strength is within self and may bring --with the attitude from the creative energies held in the active forces of self--greater relief not only for self but a marvelous relief for others." 701-1

Therefore:

"...the entity, with the very words or the blessings in planting even a nut, may insure the next generation a nut-bearing tree! The entity with its very abilities of the magnetic forces within self, may circle one with its hands and it'll bear no more fruit, though it may be bearing nuts in the present.
"These are indications, then, of how the entity may use the energies or vibrations, even of the body, constructively or destructively. Do not use these for self in either direction. For as just indicated, if you plant one, be sure it is for the next generation and not for this one. It is others ye must think of, as should every soul. 'Others, Lord, others-that I may know Thee the better.'" 3657-1

The electro-magnetic forces of the body are to be used always for the benefit of others, that is, used constructively, and not destructively. They are not only intensified by giving such magnetic treatments to others, but are also strengthened by that

positive attitude of mind and will of the individual
in his helpfulness to others.

*"Know that the body creates, or will revive
itself. Then keep the attitude of optimism and
helpfulness to others, and this will make the
same environment for self. Worry more about
somebody else than yourself and youl'll be a
lot better off."* 540-11

The positive mind and will are to the body what
the magneto is to the automobile. As the electric
sparks from the magneto ignite the gas, it thus generates the power that drives the automobile, so the
positive vibrations generated by a confident and a
determined will, create in the body those positive
electro-magnetic currents which incite and stimulate
all of the vital activities.

A teacher who possesses magnetism can easily,
if not totally subdue and control the unruliest and
incorrigible of pupils, without the use of strap or
scolding or punishment of any kind.

Many a parent has controlled a child by the mere
glance of the eye. Many a person quails and flinches
before the eye of another, as we well know.

It may be asked how the eye can convey vibratory
action to another person's eye. The answer, of course,
is this: It is the power of the WILL, the power of a
concentration of mind and will towards an objective.
It makes no difference how hardened a person may be.
For instance, an unarmed man captured by himself an
armed desperado, whom even armed police were afraid
to approach. But this man yielded to this person not
knowing why he did so; such is the power of will.

*"Yet, know that no urge, no sign, no emotion
--whether of a latent mental nature or of a
material or emotional nature finding expression in the body--surpasses that birthright,
WILL--the factor which makes the human soul,
the human individual, DIFFERENT from all other
creatures in the earth, from all manifestations of God's activity."* 2172-1

"Yet the entity, thine own soul, has been given a will to use the attributes of soul, mind and body to thine own purposes. Thus as the individual entity applies self in relationship to those facts, the entity shows itself to be a true child, or a wayward child, or a rebellious child, of the Creative Force, or God."3376-2

So:

"...With each development, that force, known upon the plane as WILL, is given to man over and above all creation; THAT force that may separate itself from its Maker, for with the WILL man may either adhere (to) or contradict the Divine law--those immutable laws, as are set between the Creator and the Created."
3744-4

Common experience teaches that the concentration of the will on the thing to be accomplished greatly enhances and increases the physical, mental, and moral powers of man.

Therefore the victory over disease is conditioned by the absolute faith, confidence, and serenity of mind on the part of the patient. The more he exercises these harmonizing and invigorating qualities of mind and will, the more favorable are the conditions for the little soldiers who are fighting his battles within his system and organs. The blood and nerve currents are less impeded and disturbed, and therefore flow more normally.

The serenity of the mind backed by absolute truth in the law and the power of a strong will, do infuse the cells and tissues with new life and vigor, thus enabling them to turn diseases into a beneficial and cleansing healing crisis.

What has just been said about the individual person, is true also of his friends and relatives.

Disease is negative. The sick person is also most exceedingly sensitive to their surroundings. And are easily influenced by all depressing, discordant, and jarring conditions. They catch expressions of fear and anxiety in the looks, the words, the gestures, and the actions of attendants, relatives, and thus intensify depressive and gloomy forebodings.

This applies especially to the influence exerted by the mother upon her ailing infant. There exists a most intimate sympathetic and telepathic connection between mother and child. The child is affected not only by the outward expression of the mother's fear and anxiety, but likewise by the doubt and despair lodged in the mother's mind and soul.

Instead of helping the disease forces destroy us we must assist the healing forces to save us by the maintaining of an attitude of absolute cheerfulness, faith, serenity and calmness. Then your looks, voice and touch will convey to the sick person the positive magnetic vibrations of health, vigor and strength. Your very presence will, therefore, radiate healing power and energy.

Herein lies the modus operandi or working basis of all successful mental and meta-physical treatments.

In the writings of meta-physical healers we often meet the assertion that they can cure organic diseases as easily and quickly as functional ailments. If they understood better the difference between functional and organic disorders they would not make such deceptive and extravagant claims. They would then realize the natural limitation of meta-physical healing.

Let us not underestimate the great value of mental, meta-physical, and spiritual healing methods. We can, however, and should aid nature's healing efforts not only by the proper mental attitude, meditation, and the prayer of faith, but also by natural living and by the many other natural methods of physical treatments that are available to all of us.

"There are many and various channels through which healing may come: Through individual contact, by faith; by laying on of hands and arousing that which will create in the mind (for it is the builder) a consciousness making for closer contact with the Universal, or Creative Force, in individual experience. Work

*the Creative Forces, in its experience...Use
that thou hast, then, in hand." 281-6*

For instance:

Mental attitude alone will not clean the house.
To concentrate on the work of house cleaning without
using broom, soap and water is not sufficient. Reason
and common sense can teach us that the removal of
physical, material encumbrances can be, to say the
least, accelerated by the use of physical or psychological agents. Anyone who has observed or who himself
experienced the efficacy of natural diet, massage and
osteopathy in dealing with the morbid accumulations
in the system, will never again underestimate the
practical value of these "brooms."

> *"So oft has this been given, and though it may
> be repeated again and again, there is only
> one way. USE THAT THOU HAST IN HAND, DAY BY
> DAY, for knowledge and understanding come with
> the application, and the experience of self
> in doing that which is known to be in accord
> with His will.*
> *"Example after example may be given in the
> experience of any individual. As they apply
> that known, knowing in whom they have believed
> with the comparisons of the ideal as the
> judgement, they come to the knowledge of the
> forces that are manifest from experience to
> experience, from day to day.*
> *"Keep that thou hast purposed, and there will
> come more and more understanding that makes
> for peace and harmony in thine experience.
> Joy comes from doing, and seeing same manifest
> in the experiences of others. Find fault in
> no one." 281-8*

> *"This is why osteopathy and hydrotherapy come
> closer to being a basis for all treatments
> needed for physical disabilities." 2524-2*

Therefore:

*"There is no form of physical mechano-therapy
so near in accord with NATURE'S measure as a
correctly given osteopathic adjustment. Others
may say what they may, but prove it by watching
those who have them regularly, and who depend
on them!"* 1158-31

*"Seek out, then, an instrument of the curative
forces known as the osteopath, that is capable
--through the proper manipulations, using the
structural portions of the body as the leverage
--of stimulating the secretions through the
various activities of glands and centers and
forces within the system itself. And we will
find that with a few adjustments--fifteen in
number, as we find, would be sufficient."* 531-2

*"Then the SCIENCE of osteopathy is not merely
the punching in a certain segment or the cracking of the bones, but it is the keeping of a
BALANCE--by the touch--between the sympathetic
and the cerebro-spinal system! THAT is real
osteopathy!*
*"With the adjustments made in this way and
manner, we will find not only helpful influences but healing with an aid to any condition
that may exist in the body--unless there is a
broken bone or the like!"* 1158-24

However:

*"Osteopathic treatments are well; but as we
have indicated, in this specific condition
these would come much later, to be of any great
help. For these corrections may be made by the
exercises of the body itself, and NATURE is
better than the osteopath--though the osteopath is the closest to the NATURAL means."*
1497-4

And massage:

"The 'why' of massage should be considered:
Inactivity cause many of those portions along
the spine from which impulses are received
to the various organs to be lax, or taut, or
allow some to receive greater impulses than
others. The massage aids the ganglia to receive
impulses from nerve forces as it aids circulation through the various portions of the
organism." 2456-4

"Well that the body, each evening, be rubbed
thoroughly with those forces as may be found
in an ointment--which acts as a lubricant for
the whole system. These may be alternated
between cocoa butter and olive oil, or olive
oil and myrrh and then cocoa butter. These
will make for bettered condition for the body's
rest and for the activities of the extremities
--as well as centers along the cerebro-spinal
system...this would also be helpful for this
body, were the spine rubbed very thoroughly,
not in the ordinary treatment as of manipulation, but a more coarseness, so that we will
stimulate the nerve ends as they function
through the muscular portion of the body."
5568-6

"At least one week out of each month should
be spent in beautifying, preserving, rectifying the body--if the body would keep young in
mind, in body, in purpose.
"This doesn't mean that the entity should spend
a whole week at nothing else. Choose three
days out of some week in each month, not just
three days in a month, but three days in some
definite week each month--either the first,
the second, the third or the fourth week of
each month--and have the general hydrotherapy
treatments, including massage, lights, and all
the treatments that are in the nature of
beautifying, and for keeping the whole of the

body-forces young.
"One week each month is required for steriliz-
ing the body functions. Then, is it any wonder
that a week after such would be well for the
supplying of the building forces for the
body's activities!" 3420-1

Hydrotherapy and Exercise:

"Hydrotherapy and physical exercise, combined
with these, should bring the better conditions
for the body. These are the manners in which
the body, or any individual body, may keep
better activities." 4003-1

Furthermore, rational mental or meta-physical
treatments support nature's efforts actively by sup-
planting the weakening and paralyzing vibrations, such
as fear, with relaxing and invigorating vibrations of
hope, confidence, and faith in the supremacy of nature's
healing forces. Under these favorable conditions, the
organism will arouse itself to the purifying and
constructive healing crises, and through these eliminate the morbid encumbrances and restore the normal
structural and functional forces.

"Know that all healing forces must be within,
not without! The applications from without
are to create within a coordinating mental
and spiritual force." 1196-7

"Know that there is within self all healing
that may be accomplished for the body. For,
all healing must come from the Divine. For
who healeth thy diseases? The source of the
universal supply. As the attitude, then, of
self, how well do ye wish to be? How well are
ye willing to cooperate, coordinate with the
Divine influences which may work in and through
thee, by stimulating the centers which have
been latent with nature's activities. For all
of these forces must come from the one source,

*and the applications are merely to stimulate
the atoms of the body. For each cell is as a
representative of a universe in itself. Then
what would ye do with thy abilities? As ye give
to others, not hating them, to know more of
the Universal Forces, so may ye have the more,
for, God is love."* 4021-1

Not only must the mechanism of the physical body
be cleansed and freed from obstructive and destructive
materials, but the injured parts must be repaired,
morbid growths and abnormal formations dissolved and
eliminated, and the lesions in the body structures
corrected by proper treatment.

*"...it is as necessary to keep the body coor-
dinating and clean as it is to keep the mental
attitude right as well as (to maintain) the
correct spiritual purposes and desires and,
most of all, keep all three consistently; and
don't be one thing in one way and another in
another way...Do right yourself, physically,
mentally and spiritually and the best will
come to you."* 5203-1

*"Often in conditions where it has been neces-
sary, you have seen unusual or abnormal strength
produced within a body, either for physical
or mental activity. Whence arose such strength?
Who hath given thee power? Within what live
ye? What is life? It is the attunement of
self, then, to the Source.*
*"How is this? When the body-physical is puri-
fied; when the mental-body is made wholly at-
one with purification or purity—with the life
and the light within itself—healing comes,
strength comes, power comes.*
*"So may an individual effect a healing, through
meditation. Not through attuning just a part
of the mind nor a portion of the body; but by
attunement of the whole to at-oneness with the
spiritual forces within—the gift of life-
force within each body."* 281-24

However:

*"Learn that the things which acquaint self
with the Divine Forces that are Creative, are
of His Making. So let the healing be accredited
to His force, wholly and entirely--even in
self, even in that that is healed.*
*"These are the First Principles, the First
Causes: all life is in Him, and self only
assists the one seeking, that he may become
aware of that Consciousness from within. For
the kingdom(with all its attributes) is within
and from within. As ye pray and meditate in
Him, so the consciousness is aroused or awakened in the experience of another, that healing
may come. For virtue--that is understanding--
must flow out of self, if healing is to be
accomplished in another." 281-10*

In organic diseases, the vitality is usually so
low, and destruction is at times so great, that the
organism cannot arouse itself to self-help. Even the
cessation of suppressive treatment and the stimulating
influence of mental or meta-physical therapeuthics is
not sufficient for bringing about the reconstructive
healing crises. This can only be accomplished by the
combined efforts and influences of all the natural
methods of living and treatment.

It is in cases like these that meta-physical
healing and hygienic living find their limitations.
Such organic defects require systematic treatment by
all the methods, active and passive, which the natural
applications can furnish. It may be slow and laborious
work to obtain, and get satisfactory results, and thus
if the vitality is too low or the destruction of the
vital parts and organs have too far advanced, even
the best and most complete combination of natural
methods of treatment may fail to produce a cure.

However, this can be determined only by a fair
trial of the natural methods. The forces of nature
are ever ready to react to persistent and systematic
efforts in the right directions; and when there is

enough vitality to keep alive, there is likely to be
enough to purify and reconstruct the organism. Time,
it is said, is the greatest healer and brings about
improvement and cure.

> *"But rather as we find, for at least another
> six months, make haste slowly; that is, keep
> very persistent and consistent with those
> applications that have been indicated for this
> body. Do not hurry through ANY of the appli-
> cations. Be as patient and as persistent in
> the daily things to be done as if the whole
> existence depended on same; for it does!"*
>
> 2606-2
>
> *"Hence with that attitude of being as persist-
> ent as the desire for indulgence, or as per-
> sistent as the devil, ye will find that ye
> bring a strength. But if ye do so doubting,
> ye are already half lost."* 1439-2

This, then, explains why, in the organic types
of disease, meta-physical methods of treatment alone
are insufficient.

CHAPTER SEVEN

WHAT IS LIFE?

In the study of the causes and characters of diseases we must endeavor to begin at the beginning, and that is life itself; for the processes of health, disease and cure are manifestation of that which we call life, vitality, energies, etc. While endeavoring to fathom the mystery of life we soon realize however, that we are dealing with an ultimate which no human mind is capable of explaining, much less solving. We can study and understand life only as it manifest, not in its origin or of its real essence.

Is life, as materialistic science claims, solely a manifestation of the electric, magnetic, and chemical activities and reactions of the physical elements composing the human organism?

Aside from inductive and deductive reasonings, the teachings as given through the Cayce readings, I find, give us the most valuable and convincing testimony on this elusive problem. They make it clear to us that the great Creative Force which animates and controls the created universe manifests as vibration in and through the forms and forces of the ascending kingdoms of nature through the four "Life Elements."

"...there are those four influences or forces in the natures of man from his source; as in environment, hereditary as of the earth and as of the mental and spiritual. These are the four corners that become represented here as the very natures or forces to which all approaches to all these influences are made in the very nature of man." 281-29

"Yet each interpretation and each application of self, of the entity, of the mental and soul mind, to its experiences in the earth, are

just as separate or distinct as may be the application of the body to the elements in the earth. EARTH, AIR, FIRE, WATER--these are one in their varied aspects, to human or bodily existence; and are each necessary." 601-11

"And remember in their combinations there are only about four elements in the body forces and yet these represent every element in the earth." 3359-1

The lowest, or mineral plane, is controlled by the electro-magnetic life element, earth; the next higher, the vegetable kingdom, by the vita-chemical life element, water; the still higher, animal kingdom, is controlled by the soul-life life element, fire; and the human kingdom by the spiritual element, air. Each of these life elements represents a higher and more refined rate of vibratory activity, and so does possess greater creative and vivifying energies or powers than the one on the lower scale.

The Edgar Cayce readings tell us that the soul force (the soul-life element) in man is part of and yet acts independently of the physical body; that after death, the soul body continues to manifest without interruption, and often acts much more vividly in the spiritual dimension. The soul-life element uses the physical and spiritual bodies as its material clothing, and as its instruments or expression in all planes of existence. It manifests in the material bodies as electricity, magnetism, nerve-force, muscle-force, thought force, etc.

"What then, the entity asks, is a soul? What does it look like? What is its plane of experience or activity? How may ye find one? It may not be separated in a material world from its own place of abode in the body-physical, yet the soul looks through the eyes of the body--it handles with the emotions of the sense of touch--it may be aware through the factors in every sense, and thus adds to its

body as much as the food of the material world has made for a growing physical body in which the soul may and does indeed dwell in its passage or activity in any individual phases of an experience in the earth." 487-17

"Many say that ye have no consciousness of having a soul--yet the very fact that ye hope, that ye have a desire for better things, the very fact that ye are able to be sorry or glad, indicates an activity of the mind that takes hold upon something that is not temporal in its nature--something that passeth not away with the last breath that is drawn but that takes hold upon the very source of its beginning--the SOUL--that which was made in the image of thy Creator." 281-41

"The SOUL is that which is the image of the Maker, and only in patience--as the Christ gave--may ye indeed become aware OF thy soul's activity; through its longings, through its convictions, through its experience into the realms of the spiritual undertakings."1348-1

Therefore:

"The body must not lose courage to carry on, but working in patience know that all healing, all help must arise from constructive thinking, constructive application and most and first of all constructive inspiration....Use (body) disturbances as stepping stones toward higher and better and greater understanding."
528-9

But medical science, as taught in the regular schools, is still dominated by the old, crude mechanical conception of Creative Force and this, as we can see, accounts for some of the gravest errors of theory and practice.

The vital conception of life, on the other hand, regards it, the primary force of all forces as coming down from the great central source of all power.

This force, which permeates, heats, and animates the entire created universe, is but the expression of the Divine Will, the "logos," the "word" of the great creative intelligence. It is this Divine Energy which sets in motion the whirls in the ether, the electricity of the corpuscles and ions that make up the different atoms and elements of matter.

These corpuscles and ions are the positive and negative forms of electricity. Electricity is a form of energy. It is intelligent energy; otherwise it could not move with the same wonderful precision within the electrons of the atoms as that of the sun and planets of the sidereal universe.

This intelligent energy can have but one source; it is but the will and the intelligence of the Creator; as Cayce expresses it, "the God-Consciousness."

> "All power, all force, is a manifestation of that which is termed the God-consciousness."
> 601-11
> "Also, in the interpretation of the universe, we find that time and space are concepts of the mental mind, as to an interpretation of or as a study into the relationships with man and to the universal or God-consciousness."
> 1747-5

If this supreme intelligence, the God-consciousness, should withdraw its energy, the electric charges (forms of energy) and with it the atoms, elements, the entire material universe would disappear as in a single momentary flash.

From this it appears that crude matter, instead of being the source of life with all its complicated mental and spiritual phenomena (which assumption, on the face of it, is absurd), is only an expression of the Life Force, itself a manifestation of the great Creative Intelligence which some call Lord, others, simply Nature, while its manifestation in man is known as the Oversoul, Superconsciousness, Brahma, Prana, etc., each term according to one's own best acceptance.

It is this supreme power and intelligence, known

as Elohim (God) and Jehovah (Lord), that are each as respectively outlined in the 1st and 2nd chapters of Genesis, acting in and through every atom, molecule, and cell in the human body, which is the true healing force, the "vis medicatrix naturæ" which is always endeavoring to repair, heal, and restore the perfection of all things. All that the physician can do, is to remove obstructions and to establish normal conditions, within and around the patient, so that "the healing force within" can do its work to its best advantage.

Here the Christian Scientist will say: "That is exactly what we claim. All is God, all is mind! There is no matter! Our attitude towards disease is based on these facts."

"Well what of it!" Suppose, in the final analysis, matter is nothing but vibration, as an expression of Divine Mind and Will. That for all practical purposes, does not justify us to deny and to therefore ignore its reality. Because I have an "all mind" body, is it advisable to place myself in the way of an "all mind" locomotive moving at the rate of sixty miles per hour?

The question is not what matter is in the final analysis, but how matter affects us. We have to be obedient to the laws of matter as we must of those of the higher planes of being, or that called spirit.

"That matter became impregnated with spirit arose from the very fact that spirit (separated) matter (or flesh) might the attributes of the source of good to be manifested." 5752-3

"That which finds itself expressed or manifested in material things is of the physical, for matter is an expression of spirit in motion to such a degree as to give the expressions in materiality.
"That which is expressed or manifested in spirit, without taking body or form, is of the spirit; yet may be manifested in the experience of an individual." 262-78

For:

"The mind of God moved, and matter, form, came into being." 262-79

"Matter began its ascent in the various forms of physical evolution in the mind of God!"
                                        262-99

Hence:

"...we find, as given that first there was for matter that gathered in a directed plane of activity called the earth, the separation of light and darkness.
"Hence these, then, are figures of that from the spiritual plane termed in the mental world as the good and evil; or in the spiritual as facing the light and the dark, or facing the source of light--which--to, the mind of those that seek to know His biddings, is the voice, the word, the life, the light, that comes in the hearts, minds, souls, of each to awaken them as individuals, to their relationships with the source of light." 262-55

CHAPTER EIGHT

LIFE IS VIBRATORY

In the final analysis, all things in nature, from a fleeting thought or emotion to the hardest piece of matter known, the diamond or platinum, are but modes of motion or vibration. Just a few years ago physical scientists assumed that an atom was one of the smallest imaginable part of a given element of matter; that although infinitesimally small it still represented solid matter. Now, in the light of the best evidence of today, we strongly suspect that there is no such thing as solid matter; that every atom is made up of charges of negative and positive electricity acting in and upon an omnipresent ether; that the difference between an atom of iron, of hydrogen, and of any other element consists solely in its number of electrical charges or corpuscles it contains, and of the velocity to which these vibrate around one another.

The Cayce readings expand on this very effectively.

"For materiality IS—or matter IS—that demonstration and manifestation of the units of positive and negative energy, or electricity, to do man's work or to destroy man himself."
412-9

"Electricity or vibration is that same energy, same power, ye call God. Not that God is an electric light or an electric machine, but vibration that is creative is of that same energy as Life itself." *2828-4*

"Life in its manifestation is vibration. Electricity is vibration. But vibration that is creative is one thing. Vibration that is destructive is another. Yet they may be from the same source." *1861-16*

"Electricity is life; life is electricity, you see. Force or the power here in the atom in itself, which is the body drawn up, we have the electric forces on the body will if given into the nervous system produce a reaction on the nerves themselves; that within, nature then produces the effect that we need to take out from the system the waste. Stimulate the body along the digestive organs, supply the force that has been burned up which should have aided the stomach in its digestion. The stomach refuses to take in the proper nourishment because it has been choked up. Ease it down; the whole system strained produces this whole effect as if it was water, too much water, but it isn't water. It is this matter being thrown in the system not being allowed to be carried off or expelled from the system."

131-1

"For as the very forces of the bodily functioning are electrical in their activity, the very action of assimilation and distribution of assimilated forces is in the physical body an active force of the very LOW yet very high VIBRATORY forces themselves." 470-22

"Whatever electricity is to man, that's what the power of God is. Man may in the material world use God-force, God-power or electricity to do man's work or to destroy man himself."

3618-1

And:

"That producing electrical units of force was just as applicable to the Universal Forces in the days of Adam as in the days of the Master, or as in the days of today." 900-70

That which is orderly, lawful, good, beautiful, natural, healthy, vibrate in unison with the harmonics of this great "Diapason of Nature"; in other words, it is alignment and attunement with the constructive principle as is found in nature, for life itself is vibratory whether manifesting in nature or in the body of man.

> "The human body is made up of electronic vibration, with each atom and element of the body, each organ and organism of same, having its electronic or unit of vibration necessary for the sustenance of, and equilibrium in that particular organism. Each unit, then, being a cell or a unit of life in itself, with its capacity of reproducing itself by the first form or law as is known of reproduction, by division of same. When any force in any organ, any element of the body, becomes deficient in its ability to reproduce that equilibrium necessary for the sustenance of the physical existence and reproduction of same, that portion becomes deficient, deficient through electronic energy as is necessary. This may become by injury, by disease, received from external forces; received from internal forces by the lack of eliminations as are reproduced in the system, by the lack of other agencies to meet the requirements of same in the body."
>
> 1800-4

Thus, the atom which was thought to be the ultimate particle of solid matter, is found to be a little universe in itself which as a corpuscle of electricity rotates or vibrates around one another like the suns and planets in the sidereal universe, very similar to the glands of the endocrine system in the human body. This explains what we mean when we say life, as energy and matter is vibratory.

As early as 1863 John Newlands discovered that when he arranged the elements of matter in the order of their atomic weight they displayed the very same relationship to one another as do the tones of the musical scale. Thus modern chemistry demonstrate the verity of the "music of the spheres," as another one of the visionary concept of ancient Mysticism. So the atoms in itself, as well as all of the atoms of matter

in relationship to one another, are constructed and
arranged in exact correspondence with the laws of order
and harmony.

"As we may see in a functioning physical
organism, electricity in its incipiency or
lowest form is the nearest vibration in a
physical sense to Life itself; for it is the
nucleus about each atom of active force or
principle set by the atomic activity of blood
pulsation itself, that begins from very union
of the plasm that creates life itself in a
physical organism. These are continued
throughout the activity of a physical body,
known and called plasms of cellular force in
the blood stream itself, building in the
various organisms of the system through the
activity of the glands or the little engines
of activity that create for the system that
necessary plasm which has gone to make for
not only the functioning of the liver but that
which would replace the liver itself; that
which would not only make for the functioning
of the kidney but that which would make for
the plasm that would rebuild the kidney itself;
not only that which supplies the pulsation and
activity of the heart but that which will also
aid to the system that which will rebuild,
replenishing the walls of the heart itself;
not only that which adds to the system and
makes for the pulsation or flow of plasm
through the nerve energy, but rebuilds the
walls of the cells that hold the plasm that
functions in its activity as nerve impulses
through the system, whether to a ganglia that
may be received from within pulsation that may
be started from without, which we know as a
reaction to the functionings of, the system's
responses to, vibration without and within;
enabling the brain to see, the brain to hear,
the brain to feel! and yet, from what source
does this arise?" 3950-1

The question naturally arising here is, "normal or abnormal with what source?" To this we would answer that the vibratory conditions of the organism must be in harmony with nature's established harmonies in the physical, mental, moral, spiritual and psychical realms of the life and action of man.

For that which is disorderly, abnormal, ugly, unnatural and unhealthy, vibrates in discord with the harmonies of nature. It is that alignment with the "Destructive Principle" in nature. It is called the beautiful and balanced order in inanimate nature for it plays in tune with the musical score of the great symphony of life. Man alone can play out of tune. This is his privilege, if he so chooses, by virtue of that freedom of choice, will and action. We can now, therefore, better understand the definitions of the principles of health as found in the catechism of nature and the readings of Cayce.

As for example:

"If you desire a robust, healthy, strong body, then think health and you will bring health. Should you weaken within yourself and feel that the physical is below normal, and you become oppressed by it, the mere suggestion causes the condition to become active within the body."
"As the entity thinketh within, so is the entity; as the spirit moves to bring about the correct physical and mental attitude towards yourself, so will it be brought." 900-254

"In the eliminations of the system physically, these are often disturbed by the accumulation of drosses as are produced; not so much by the physical inactivity of organs or of the active forces in the functioning of the system, as of the mental destructive forces created by worry. Worry and fear being, then, the greatest foes to normal healthy physical body, turning the assimilated forces in the system

into poisons that must be eliminated, rather
than into life giving vital forces for a
physical body." 5497-1

Let us see whether we can make this clear by a
simile. If a timepiece is in excellent condition, "in
harmonious vibration," its movement is then adjusted
so as to coincide exactly, in point of time with the
rotations of the earth around its axis. The established
regular movement of the earth forms the basis of the
established harmonious relationship between the vibrations of a normal and "healthy" time-piece and the
revolutions of our planet. The watch has to vibrate
in unison with the harmonics of the planetary universe
in order to be normal, or in harmony.

In like manner, everything that is good, natural,
healthy, normal, beautiful, must vibrate in unison
with its correlated harmonics in Nature.

"He should remember, in making a study, while
life is an electrical energy, there are
vibrations of the nature in the system, All
disorders as set themselves up in a body, by
correlating of their individual vibrations,
create a specific disturbance. Not all of
galvanic nor all of any one type of electrical
vibrations then are set up in the varied
disturbances, but all types are indicated. And
there are those that are constructive to
certain vibrations, there are those that are
destructive. There are those vibrations that
will enable organs to be aroused to an activity.
There are those that would destroy the acti-
vity of organs, whether these are in accord
with the general system or to that balance to
which the body is best adapted in itself.
"These then should be studied, and know that
constructive are the lowest forms, destructive
the higher forms." 1249-1

The Edgar Cayce philosophy presents a rational
concept of evil, of its causes and purposes, namely:

that it is brought on by violation of nature's laws; that it is destructive in its purposes; that it can be overcome only by compliance with the law. There is no suffering, disease, or evil of any kind anywhere unless the law has been transgressed somewhere, sometime by someone.

These transgressions of the law may be due to ignorance, to indifference, or to wilfulness and viciousness. The effects will always commensurate with the cause.

The science of natural healing and living shows clearly that what is called disease is primarily the efforts of nature to eliminate morbid matter and to restore the normal functions of the body; that the processes of disease are just as orderly in their own way as everything else in nature; that we must not check or suppress symptoms but cooperate with them to learn their origination. Thus we can, slowly and laboriously, learn the all-important lesson that "obedience to the law" is the only means of preventing disease, and is thereby, of course, the only true cure.

> "Learn the LAW; that ye reap what ye sow! The manner in which ye measure to others, it will be measured to thee again! That is an unchangeable law!
> "Then, live the law; be the law, as respecting such." 2185-1

> "Rather that as builded, does the meriting of same--in the application of the laws as pertain to universal forces--become the law in the individual's activity. Be rather the law, than within the law, or conforming to a law. Be a law." 1729-1

> "For it is the law to BE the law, and the LAW is love!" 1158-9

Therefore:

> "...when the law is coordinated, in spirit,

in mind, in body, the entity is capable of fulfilling the purpose for which it enters a material or physical experience." 2528-2

"There must be a law to EVERYTHING--spirit, mental, material. To be sure, there IS; but it is guided, guarded, watched over, and kept in accord with that which is the principle, the spirit, the soul of the First Cause."
1885-2

Also:

"It is not all for an entity, or a soul, to have knowledge concerning law; whether karmic law, spiritual law, penal law, social law, or whatnot. The condition is, what does the entity do ABOUT the knowledge that is gained! Is the knowledge used to evade cause and effect, or is it used to coerce individuals into adhering to the thoughts of self? or is it used to aid others in their understanding of the law, and thus bring the cause to that position where the will of the Creative influence is supreme; or the power that comes with making the will one with the law of love, of karma, of cause and effect, of every influence--one with Creation!
342-2

The fundamental laws of healing, cause and effect, action and reaction, as revealed by the Cayce readings, impressed upon me the truth that there is nothing accidental or arbitrary in the processes of health, disease and cure; that every changing condition is either in harmony or in discord with the order of the universe and the laws of our being; that only by complete surrender and obedience to the law can we attain and maintain perfect health and happiness.

Thus the readings bring home to us constantly and forcibly the inexorable facts of natural law and the necessity of being in compliance with the law. Herein lies the great educational, moral value to the individual and to the race itself. The man who has learned to master his bad habits and his voracious appetites, so as to conform with nature's laws on the physical plane, and who has thereby regained his bodily health, realizes that personal effort and self-control are the master key to all further development on the mental and spiritual planes of being. That self-mastery and unremitting and unselfish personal effort are the only means of self-completion for individuals as well as social salvation.

The individual who has regained his health and strength through obedience to the laws of his being, enjoys a measure of self-content, gladness of soul, and enthusiasm which cannot be explained by the mere possession of physical health. These highest and purest attainments of the human soul are not the results of mere physical well-being, but of the peace and harmony which come only from obedience to the law. Such is "the peace of God, which passeth all understanding."

"The whole of God's creation seeks harmony and peace! So, the desire of the soul for harmony and peace is born of Him that gave, 'My peace I give unto thee'; not as the world gives peace, but as the spirit that makes alive, that which gives the knowledge of His peace-- that peace that passeth all understanding."

1742-4

CHAPTER NINE

SUGGESTIVE AFFIRMATIONS

Suggestive affirmations of health are justified in the face of disease. The health conditions must be first established in the mind before they are conveyed to and impressed upon all of the atoms of the body.

The well-being of the physical body as a whole depends upon the health of each of the billions of minute atoms which comprises the body. These atoms are so small that they have to be magnified several hundred times under a powerful microscope before any of them can be seen.

> *"Each and every atom in the human body is a world in itself, and with the grand central forces of self in a perfect onement there is given every effort towards making perfection in every atom of the body. These becoming hindered by any influence, it either builds or breaks the will of that atomic force, and is as the same as may be applied in an individual life, raised to an Nth degree. See?*
>
> 136-63
>
> *"As we have in the body of a living physical being, we have a body made up of many atoms, and their relations to each other depends upon the force as is given in each part..."* 3744-2

> *"Each atom of the body-physical is an expression of a spiritual import. That is how matter comes into being. That through rebellious forces within an atomic structure portions become as warriors against good, as set up within a physical body, is proven by dis-ease and distress, both mental and physical."*
>
> 264-45

Much of the work of an army is carried out on

through different, well-established departments, as the commissariat, the hospital service, the air force, infantry, etc. Though the life and the activities of the army are so well regulated that they almost seem automatic, nevertheless much depends upon the leader or commander-in-chief.

The vital processes of the physical organism, digestion, assimilation, elimination, respiration, the circulation of the blood, etc., are going on without our conscious volition, whether we be awake or asleep. These involuntary activities are impelled by the sympathetic nervous system, while the voluntary functions of the body are controlled through the motor nervous system. This division, however, is not a sharp one, and the two departments frequently overlap one another.

The cerebro-spinal system resembles the commissarial department of the army, which attends to the material welfare of the soldiers, while the sympathetic system, with headquarters in the brain, corresponds to the commander with his executive staff, the nerve centers in the spinal cord and other parts of the body being subordinate officers in the field.

While the physical well-being of the army depends almost entirely upon the automatic work of its different departments, its mind and soul is the man leading it. He determines the spirit, the energy as well as the efficiency of this vast organization.

The marvellous work performed by these little cellular organisms, as well as observations made in the dissecting room and under the microscope, strongly indicate that these cells are endowed with some sort of individual intelligence. They do their work without our aid or conscious volition. But, nevertheless, are greatly influenced by the varying conditions of the mind. While their activities seem to be controlled through the sympathetic nervous system, they stand in direct telegraphic communication with "headquaters" in the brain where every impulse of the mind is conveyed to them.

"That portion of the body, better known as the

*one that propagates or takes care of the body
--physical, mental, moral or whatnot, when it
is not able to take care of itself.*
*"SUB-CONSCIOUS IS UNCONSCIOUS force. This may
be seen in every nerve end, in every muscular
force. Subconscious action may be brought
into manifestation by the continual doing of
certain acts in this physical plane, so the
body becomes unconscious of doing the acts
that it does."* 3744-1

If there be dismay and confusion in the mind,
this condition is telegraphically conveyed over nerve
trunks and filaments to every cell in the body, and
as a result these little workers and soldiers become
panic-stricken and are hence incapable of rightly
performing their manifold duties.
The cell system of the body resembles a vast
army. The mind is the general at the head of it. The
cells are the soldiers, divided into different and
numerous groups to do any special work required.

*"In the make-up of the active forces of the
physical body, it is constituted of many, many
cells--each with its individual world within
itself, controlled by the spirit that is ever-
lasting, and guided by that of the soul, which
is a counterpart..."* 5756-4

*"Then, the activities of the will, the con-
sciousness, the various terms that have been
and are applied to the manner of expression
in consciousness are the basic thoughts, the
basic activities through which each should
prepare self for the abilities, for the acti-
vating forces that may assist self..."* 262-40

*"As has been given, certain forces in the
system are the channels through which activa-
ting sensations rise; for transmission to
portions of the physical body which act to
send out vibrations for healing. The (pumping)*

sensations, then, are but the samples--the attempts of those forces to rise and become active in the consciousness of the body. Do not force them; but so conduct the mind's trend and the body's activities as to leave self a channel for such expression." 281-12

Therefore, if the commander-in-chief lacks the insight, force, and determination, the discipline of the army will be very lax, and its efficiency greatly impaired. If he is craven, without faith in himself and in the cause he represents, his lack of courage, his doubts and indecisions, and especially his fears, will thereby communicate or transmit themselves to the entire army, resulting in its discouragement and total defeat.

"The fears in the experience of any individual or entity are the losing hold upon that as to WHO is able to supply the strength, the courage, the aid necessary." 954-4

"Know, however, that...what the will does about what is set as its ideal--in mental and material as well as spiritual experiences-- and then having the courage to carry out that ideal; this makes the difference, between constructive and creative relationships, and those that make one rather a drifter, or ne'er- do-well, or one very unstable and unhappy."
1401-1

Therefore, the most successful commanders have been those who were possessed of absolute confidence in themselves and in the efficiency of their army, who in the face of gravest danger and discouraging situations pressed on to the predetermined goal with doggedness and courage and resolution. Determination and pertinacity of this kind create the magnetic power which imparts itself to every individual soldier in the army and makes him a willing subject, even unto the death, to the will of his commander.

> *"There is no urge in the astrological, in the*
> *vocational, in the hereditary or the environ-*
> *mental—which surpasses the will or determi-*
> *nation of an entity..." 5023-2*

When the pest was invading Napoleon's army, that great general entered the hospitals where the victims of the plague were lying, took them by the hand, and conversed with them. He did this to overcome the fear in the hearts of his soldiers, and thus to protect them against the dread disease. He said, "A man whose will can conquer the world, can conquer the plague."

To my mind, this was one of the greatest deeds of the Corsican General. At a time when such ideas were practically unknown, the genuis of this man had so grasped its principles, he was making them factors in his apparent success. "Apparent" because, while we admire his genuis, we deplore the ends to which he finally applied his wonderful powers.

At times when the battle seemed lost, Napoleon would go to the front where the danger was the greatest, for by the mere sight of him the hard-pressed soldiers under his command were inspired to superhuman effort and thereby achieved an easy victory.

As long as the glamor of invincibility surrounded him, Napoleon was invincible, because he infused into his soldiers a faith and courage which nothing could withstand. But when the cunning of the Russian bear broke his power and decimated his ranks on the ice-bound "steppes," the hypnotic spell was broken also. Friends and enemies alike recognized that, after all, he was but a man, subject to chance and circumstance; and from that time on he was vulnerable and suffered defeat after defeat.

The power of the mind over the physical body and its involuntary functions (the functions which are regulated and controlled through the sympathetic nervous system) may be illustrated by the demonstrable facts of hypnotism. Through the exertion of his own imagination and his will-power, the hypnotist can so dominate the brain, and through the mind the physical body of his subject, as to influence not only the sensory functions, but also affect heart action and respiration. By the power of his will the hypnotist is able to retard or accelerate pulse and respiration, even to subdue the heart beat so that it becomes and is hardly perceptible.

If it is possible thus to control by the power of will the vital functions in the body of another person, it must be possible to also control those functions in our own bodies. Many yogis and fakirs have developed this power of the mind over the physical body to a marvelous extent.

Herein lies the true domain of mental therapeutics. We can learn to dominate and regulate the vital activities and the life currents in our bodies so that they carry out their work intelligently and harmoniously even under the stress of illness and danger. We can, by the power of will direct the vital currents to those parts and organs which need them most, and therefore, relieve congested areas by equalizing or increasing the circulation, and by drawing from the surplus of blood and nerve currents and distributing the vital force over other parts of the body that are lacking this energy.

Such was the case of the young Edgar Cayce who had lost his voice and the doctors could not restore it by any means. This impedement lasted for over one year until someone suggested that hypnosis be used, where finally the suggestion was given him to increase the blood supply to the throat area, effecting a cure. And from this initial incident began the Edgar Cayce legacy that is of benefit to so many people.

"All force controlling any individual body is reached by suggestion to the physical, soul or spiritual forces. By suggestion we mean: Saying a thing is black, it is black; saying a thing is wet, it is wet, etc. To this body here, say to it that it will become normal in its waking state; that the circulation will be so equalized as to remove strain from any and every part of the body. Just to say, "You are not going to have any headaches when you

wake up," doesn't mean anything." 294-4

"All bodies are amenable to suggestion through the abnormal mind, or through the subconscious mind, or through the sympathetic nerve system of the body." 4648-2

Therefore:

"...would be well that suggestion for self and through self be impressed upon the developing body sufficient that the sympathetic, with the cerebro-spinal, may coordinate in the whole with the sensory system." 4223-2

Also:

"...each organ, each gland of the system, receives impulses through this manner for its activity.
"Hence we find there are reactions to every portion of the system by suggestion, mentally, and by the environment and surroundings."
1158-24
"Just as the suggestions may be used that have been made to the body through some of the treatments outlined--the mind acts upon the resuscitating forces of the physical being, by and through suggestion. Just so there may be the realization that spiritual forces are a part of the whole physical being." 1992-3

We must be careful, however, to use our higher powers in conformity with nature's intent; that is, we must not endeavor to suppress nature's cleansing and healing efforts. It is possible to do this by the power of will as well as with drugs or with the giving of wrong suggestions.

"So when the psychic forces are not abused, but are used properly they assist. When they are abused by wrong conditions, by wrong

suggestions, or by seeking wrong information (EC), they bring stress and strain." 294-55

"Suggestions to the conscious mind only brings to the mental plane those forces that are of the same character and the conscious is the suggestion in action. In that of suggestion to the unconscious mind, it gives its reflection or reaction from the universal forces or mind or superconscious forces. By the suggestion just as given may be wavered by the forces that are brought to bear on the subconscious to reach the conscious mind, just as we have in a purely mechanical form." 3744-2

Mentally and emotionally, as well as physically, we must work with nature, not against her, and when we understand all the fundamental laws of suggestive affirmations in the disease and healing process, we cannot but well do otherwise.

"In directing the body, then, either verbally or in the undertone or in the desire of all present, make the affirmation that only the highest may guide in all experiences; and there will grow the more perfect attunement by the associations of that consciousness ever of those present. And be they saint or sinner, rich or poor, stranger and closest in association, they should ever be asked to hold that affirmation through every period of laying aside the conscious self to enter in communication with the highest that may be attained in self. And those who cannot conform should not be present." 254-73

In the above lies another key, affirmations, for the prevention of disease, physically, emotionally and mentally, as well as letting the highest in us be the guide in our everyday living.

Therefore:

"...each affirmation should, and does, fill a place, a purpose, in the minds, in the hearts of those that--through concerted and consecrated effort--seek to be a channel and to be one with Him." 281-26

"In the consideration of such affirmations, would be well that each be given or repeat that which raises for self, or those being aided, that which arouses the consciousness for the individual, rather than too general an one; but this one that would cover all:
"THERE IS BEING RAISED WITHIN ME THAT CHRIST CONSCIOUSNESS THAT IS SUFFICIENT FOR EVERY NEED WITHIN MY BODY, MY MIND, MY SOUL." 281-7

The new holistic psychology and the science of mental and spiritual healing teach us that the lower principles in man stand or should stand under that guidance of the higher. The physical body, with its material elements, should not be dominated but guided by the mental and the spiritual. The mind is inspired through the inner consciousness, which is the source of all life and all intelligence animating the human organism.

Wherever this natural order is reversed, there is discord or disease. Too many people think and act as though the physical body alone were all in all, as though it were the only thing worth caring for and thinking about. They exaggerate the importance of the physical to the detriment of the mental and of the spiritual and, therefore, become abject slaves to the material elements only.

The physical body is the lowest and the least intelligent of the different principles that make up the human entity. Yet people allow their minds and their souls to become dominated and terrified by the sensations of the physical body.

When the servants in the house so control and so terrify the master, when the master becomes the slave and do with him as they please, there cannot be order and harmony in that house.

We may expect the same results when the lower principles in man lord it over the higher. When physical weakness, illness, and pain fill the mind with fear and dismay, reason becomes clouded, the will atrophies, and self-control is lost.

Every thought and every emotion has its direct effect upon the physical constituents of the body. The mental and emotional vibrations become physical counterparts and structures. Discord in the mind is translated into physical disease in the body, while the harmonies of hope, faith, cheerfulness, happiness, love, and altruism create in the organism the corresponding health vibrations.

"And know the physical result is first conceived in spirit, acted upon by mind, and then manifested in the material--with what spirit ye entertain." 2813-1

"The spiritual is the life, the mental is the builder, the material is the result of that builded through the purposes held by the individual entity." 622-6

"Remember, as ye do this, that which has been given; the spirit maketh alive, the mind is the builder, the application is the experience in the individual life." 262-119

It has been proved over and over again by everyday experience that mental and emotional conditions positively affect the chemical composition of the tissues and secretions of the body. The destructive emotions of fear, worry, anger, revengefulness, envy and jealousy, actually poison the fluids and tissues of the body. The bite of an angry man may cause blood poisoning, and prove as fatal as the bite of a mad dog. It creates within the body a number of poisonous secretions.

Therefore:

"The mind, through anger, may make the body do
that which is contrary to the better influence
of same; it may make for a change in its
environ, its surrounding, contrary to the laws
of environment or hereditary forces that are
a portion of the 'elan vitale' of each manifested body, with the spirit or the soul of
the individual." 3645-17

"Anger causes poisons to be secreted by the
glands (adrenals principally). Joy has the
opposite effect." 281-54

"Anger may upset the body and cause a great
deal of disturbance, to others as well as self."
3621-1

"For anger can destroy the brain as well as
any disease. For it is itself a disease of the
mind." 3510-1

However:

"It is well that anger and its ability for
expression be existent, but woe to those who
allow same to become stumblingblocks, and to
cause hate, malice and injustice to be dealt
in ANY manner to their fellow man!" 2132-1

"Hence those influences that make for the
expressions in anger should be much as may
have been said by some, 'When anger arises,
at least count ten before you speak,' that
will save not only self but many regrets and
many associations that are for a greater and
more satisfactory experience in this particular sojourn." 1003-2

"The entity may be mad and sin not. Righteous
anger is a virtue. He that has no temper is
very weak, but he that controls not his temper
is much worse. That ye experience in thy
activities at times. This is active patience.

Don't think it, much less do it. For as the man thinketh in his heart, so is he." 3416-1

"Poor indeed is he who does not ever show anger, but worse is he who cannot control it in himself. And there most fail. Though often those who flare up quickly, also forgive quickly--if they remain as little children asking, seeking, living, 'Guide thou me, O God, in the steps I take and in the words I say day by day.'" 3645-1

Fear is one of the most destructive emotions known and it does affect each one of us every single day of the year. It is the cause of so many hardships and ailments. The list is never ending.

"For fear is--as it ever has been--that influence that opposes will, and yet fear is only of the moment while will is of eternity. Hence fear takes hold upon the emotions, while will is deeper-seated into the soul, into the warp and woof of the very being of an entity in its entirety; finding expression to be sure in the lowest of the emotions, yet it is prompted by the creative force itself." 1210-1

"Fear creates doubt. Doubt brings such conditions in which the spirit becomes weak, and the material seems to take first place. Yet these are not in keeping with the tenets nor the intent of the individual.... So, as ye have found, so as ye may find in thy experiences in the present, doubt and fear are cast away when the thoughts are lifted to the hope that comes in the Cross, even in the cross of Jesus."
                                                2272-1

Therefore:

"Fear is the root of most of the ills of mankind whether of self, or of what others think of self, or what self will appear to

*others. To overcome fear is to fill the mental,
spiritual being with that which wholly casts
out fear..." 5459-3*

*"In thine own heart there comes those things
that would make afraid. But fear is of the
earth. The spirit of truth and righteousness
casteth out fear." 397-1*

Sudden fear, as anger, or any other destructive
emotion in the nursing mother may cause illness or
even death of the infant. Such are the powers of the
emotions upon the physical body.

In psychological laboratories it has been found
by scientifically conducted experiments that persons
under the influence of destructive mental and emotional
conditions the secretions and excretions of the body
show an increase of morbid and poisonous elements.

Selfishness, anger, and worry contract and congeal
the blood vessels, the nerve fibers, the channels of
the endocrine system, through which the life forces
are conveyed from the innermost source of life to the
different parts and organs of the body. The flow of
the life currents is impeded and diminished. Such are
the actual physiological effects of fear, anxiety,
and egotism on the physical organism.

*"These arise from the creative center of the
body itself, and as they go through the various
centers direct same; else they may become
greater disturbing than helpful. Surround self
with that purpose, 'Not my will, O God, but
thine be done, ever.' and the entity will
gain vision, perception and--most of all
judgement." 2623-3*

A man under the influence of great fear as one
exposed to freezing temperatures present the very same
outward appearance, so may death result in both through
the congealing of the tissues and the shutting out of
the life currents. The person afflicted with the worry
habit may not die suddenly like the one overcome with

great and sudden fear. Nevertheless, fear and worry vibrations maintained constantly will surely obstruct and diminish the inflow of the life force, lower the vitality and therewith increase the non-resistance and the encroachment of influences inimical to the health of the individual organism.

The cells in the body are negative, or, at least, they should be negative in relationship to the positive mind. The relationship of the mind to the cell should be like that of hypnotist to subject. If the mind could not exert such absolute control over the cells and organs as cell groups, it would be impossible for us to walk, talk, write, dodge danger, etc., with almost automatic ease.

The cells are not able to reason upon the truth or untruth of the suggestion conveyed to them from the mind within or an individual mind without. They accept the promptings unqualifiedly and act accordingly.

Thus, if the mind constantly thinks of, say, the stomach as being in badly diseased condition, unable to do its work properly, the mental images of weakness and disease with their accompanying fear vibrations are telegraphed over the efferent nerves to the cells of the stomach, and these become more and more weakened and distressed through the destructive vibrations as sent to them from the mind.

I often consult a book on anatomy and physiology to study and to keep constantly before the mind's eye the normal structure and functions of a healthy liver or stomach, or whatever organ may be of interest at the present moment. This, of course, now brings to the fore the power of visualization.

CHAPTER TEN

VISUALIZATION

Many books have been written expounding the powers of visualization. There are as many techniques as there are authors. However, the Edgar Cayce readings are most explicit on this very interesting discipline.

> *"The visualizing of any desire as may be held by an individual will come to pass, with the individual acting in the manner as the desire is held. The manners in which this entity is going about the visualizations are well. We would not alter them save in that these be not forced upon anyone that has not had some vision of his own--see?"* 311-6

Seeing the corrections to be desired within the mental will create the accomplishment in the body.

> *"Remembering that the mental is the Builder. See self with the added forces necessary for the correction, as well and strong and revibrating to the new flood of blood and energy as is being created in the system by the proper vibrations being set up in the physical body, and we will find the body will respond and build that image held before its inner self. Do that."* 5642-5

> *"While these are active in the system, well that there be kept that continued attitude of seeing the body replenished, rebuilded, in a mental, a spiritual, and a material way and manner. This held by the body-consciousness as seeing these things accomplished will aid also in the correcting in the physical forces of the body."* 4482-1

"For the body is able within itself to see those activities taking place, will there be given or known that which is being desired to be accomplished in the body, see? Get that! That's the differentiation--able to be seen and known by the body-functioning and body activities itself." 1742-3

Also:

"In the activities of the mind of man, a visualization is a portion of a material experience, no matter whether in the present experience or a combination and correlation of many experiences. While that felt is the sum total of all experiences, correlated with the superconscious, or the life itself, provided the purport of the individual is in keeping with the purport of life, or truth, see? Then we find when one--as the body here, my servant (137) visualizes this the sum of the experience, but of the divine--hence, as has oft been said, those that would guide the body--mentally, physically and spiritually--are above the normal or ordinary, or the regular--or the even higher forces in cosmic influence. Hence harder to visualize until felt. When felt, the visualization is a portion of the activity set out." 900-422

"Hence the body should be able, with a little visualization of that as is desired by the self, to create for itself that atmosphere, that environ, for that being acted upon! This requires the necessary knowledge of the body, of the mind, of that as is desired by the body. Then with that knowledge and the proper visualization, the understanding comes." 1048-3

In the understanding of the power of visualization, we can also direct positive vibrations to many others that are in need of help.

"As the vibrations are raised within self through this very visualization, then experiencing of there being the activities, the body --as everyone--is able to send, or direct, or create an environ--to such an one to whom the thought is directed--that is helpful, hopeful, beneficial in every way." 281-15

"By visualizing in such manners those meditations that are given out for others, for self; for in aiding others does one aid one's self most. And unless this is so visualized from without self, it becomes rote. But when made, set, or so experienced by the inner self as being an active, living principle within self, it ceases to become rote." 281-15

However, the following guidance is given in the Edgar Cayce readings, and needs to be considered when visualizing. This question was asked of Cayce:

"Q.- To bring a desired thing or condition into manifestation, is it advisable to visualize it by making a picture or just to hold the idea in prayer and let God produce it in His own way without our making a pattern?
"A.- The Pattern is given thee in the mount. The mount is within thine inner self. To visualize by picturing is to become idol worshippers. Is this pleasing, with thy conception of thy God that has given, 'Have no other gods before me'? The god in self, the God of the universe, then, meets thee in thine inner self. Be patient, and leave it with Him. He knoweth that thou hast need of before ye ask. Visualizing is telling Him how it must look when you have received it. Is that thy conception of an All-Wise, All-Merciful Creator? Then, let rather thy service ever be, 'Not my will, O God, but Thine be done in me, through me. For all is His.' Then, think like it--and most of all, act like it is." 705-2

Therefore:

"Visualize not as of that in the picturization,
but rather visualize as in the tones of music
that may give tones in color, in painting or
picture of the Christ Consciousness in self.
This will raise self more and more to the
greater abilities in self in every direction."
                                        275-37

Have you ever noticed how the written or printed notes of a tone piece or the perforation on the paper music roll of an automatic piano player are arranged in symmetrical and geometrical figures and groups? Dry sand strewn on the top of a piano on which harmonious tone combinations are produced, shows a tendency to arrange itself in symmetrical patterns.

In this you have a visual illustration of the translation of harmonious sound vibrations, which express "the harmonics of the soul's emotions," into correspondingly harmonious arrangements and configurations in the physical material of the paper roll.

A jumble of discords of sound, if reproduced on a music roll, would represent a chaotic jumbles of perforations.

Thus the purely mental and emotional is translated into its corresponding discords or harmonics in the physical reality.

As the perforations on the paper music roll arrange themselves either symmetrically or without symmetry and order, in strict accordance with the harmonics or discords of the composition, so the atoms, molecules, and cells in the physical body group themselves in normal or abnormal structures of health or of disease in exact correspondence with the harmonics or the discordant vibrations conveyed to them from the mental and emotional planes.

"For, vibrations take color and tone--as does
a personality of one individual to another."
                                        294-204
"For of course the tonal vibration is that
which produces color...color and tone   are

just different rates of vibration." 2779-1

"...sounds, music and colors may have much to do with creating the proper vibrations about individuals that are mentally unbalanced, physically deficient or ill in body or mind..."
                                           1334-1

Another illustration: Two violins, as they leave the shop of the maker, are exactly alike in material, structure, and quality tone. One of the two stringed instruments is constantly used by beginners and by persons incapable of producing pure notes. The other passes into the hand of an artist who understands how to use the instrument to the best advantage and who draws from it only musical tones that are true in pitch and tone quality.

After a few years, compare the two violins again. You will find that the one used by the tyros in music has deteriorated in its musical qualities, while the one in the hands of the artist has greatly improved in quality and purity of tone. What is the reason? The atoms and molecules in the wood of the two instruments have grouped themselves according to the discords or the harmonies that have been produced from them.

If this arrangement of molecules is possible in supposedly "dead wood," how much easier must be this adjustment of atoms, molecules, and cells to discordant or harmonious vibratory influence in the "living," plastic and fluidic human organism.

What harmony is to music, hope, faith, happiness, cheerfulness, sympathy, love, and altruism are to the vibratory conditions of the human entity. These emotions are in alignment with the constructive principle in nature. They "harmonize" the physical vibrations, relax the tissues, and open them wide to the inflow. of the life forces.

"The body is supersensitive to vibrations, whether they be of light, color, or motion; all of which, of course, in essense are one, yet find their manifestations in varied degrees; which applied in the experience of

an individual may at times, as in this indi-
vidual at times, bring periods when too much
of the one has made for an unbalancing in the
physical reactions in the other direction."

1770-1

Swedenborg truly says: "The warmth of life is in
the heat of the divine love permeating and animating
the universe." The more we posses of hope, faith love,
and their kindred emotions, the more we open ourselves
to the inflow and action of the vital energies. The
good-natured, cheerful, lovable, sympathetic person
is found to be "more alive" than the crabbed, morose,
selfish individual.

"The body is spiritual in its aspects and its
reactions. If the body will aid self in those
applications as may be made for same, see self
--in periods when the body enters into the
quiet--healed as it, the body, would be
healed. Vision self being aided by those
applications. Know what each application is
for, seeing that doing that within self. Keep
the mind in that attitude as makes for conti-
nuity of forces manifesting through self--a
continual flow, see?" 326-1

"Those vibrations as may be had by the concerted
activity of individuals, that may be able to
raise their own imaginative (if so chosen to
be called) forces within self, to see those
activities taking place within the active
forces of the body, (5576), we will find this
will also aid. Seek and ye shall find; knock
and it will be opened! See that being accom-
plished, and it will aid much." 5576-1

"Be oft in prayer, oft in meditation, seeing
self gaining the proper nourishment, proper
resuscitating forces from those elements being
given to the system for its resuscitation."

2097-1

CHAPTER ELEVEN

VITALITY

One of the first primary causes of disease, is lowered vitality. What can we do to increase vitality? Old school physicians and most people in general seem to think that this can be done by consuming large quantities of nourishment, food or drink, and by the use of stimulants and health tonics.

The constant cry of patients is: "Doctor, if you could only prescribe some good tonic or some pills that will give me strength, then I should be all right! I am sure that this is all I need to be cured."

We all fully agree with the patient's need for more vitality to overcome disease, but unfortunately this cannot be obtained only from food and drink, or from stimulants and tonics.

"Vitality," Life Energy or Life Force, whatever it may be called or whatever its aspect, is something that we cannot eat or drink. It is independent of the body and of material food. If the body should so fall "dead," the so called life force would still continue to act just as vigorously in the spiritual body, which is the exact counterpart of the physical organism.

The physical-material body as well as the spiritual-material body are only the instruments for the manifestation of the life force. For they are no more "life" itself than the violin is to the artist.

But just as the violin must be kept in excellent or best condition in order to enable the artist to draw from it the harmonies of sound, so food and drink are necessary to keep the physical body in the best possible condition for the manifestation of vital force. The more normal the physical and spiritual bodies are in structure and function, the more harmonious our thought forms and emotional life; the more abundant will be the influx of vital force into the organism and its many functional parts.

110

*"Keep a normal—NORMAL physical activity, as
to diet, as to the health rules and regulations.
ALL of these are better than all of those drawn
from fanciful combinations that wreck portions
of the body." 1158-17*

*"Live and keep normal activities. Begin with
the study of self—not anatomically but
spiritually. And the greater spiritual lesson
you may gain is in the 5th chapter of Matthew.
Learn this by heart, then read the 14th chapter
of John and the 12th chapter of Romans. Then
live them." 3364-1*

Therefore:

*"Do not be excessive in anything! Do not be
abnormal! Let's be normal in everything!"*
                                    340-29

Ignorance of these simple truths leads to the
most serious mistakes. Physicians and people in general
do not stop to think that excessive drinking as well as
wrong thinking, tends to rob the body of the necessary
vitality instead of supplying it.

The processes of digestion, assimilation, and
elimination of food and drink in themselves require
a considerable expenditure of vital force. Therefore,
all foods taken in excess of the actual needs of the
body consumes life force that should be available for
other purposes, as for the execution of physical and
mental work.

The Romans had a good proverb: "Plenus venter non
studet libenter"--"A full stomach does not like to
study." The most wholesome foods, if taken in excess,
will clog the system with waste matter just like too
much coal will dampen and extinguish the fire burning
in the furnace creating a residue of clunkers.

Furthermore, the morbid materials and systemic
poisons produced by impure, unsuitable, and wrongly
combined foods will clog the cells and tissues of the
body, cause unnecessary frictions, and obstruct the
inflow and operation of vital energies, just as dust

in a watch will clog and impede the movements of its
inner mechanism.

> *"Keep an even, normal balance in diet of body,*
> *diet of mind, and the use and associations of*
> *same in every way; for as a man thinketh in*
> *his heart (not as he speaks, but as he thinketh*
> *in his heart) so is he. So, keep the body fit,*
> *keep the mind fit. Do not allow little anta-*
> *gonisms of the body or mind to undo thou hast*
> *builded in thine experience." 257-136*

The greatest artist living cannot draw harmonious
sounds from the strings of the finest "Stradivarius"
if the body of the violin is filled with fine dust
particles. Likewise, the life force cannot act any more
perfectly in a body filled with morbid encumbrances.

The human organism is capable of liberating and
manifesting daily a limited quantity of vital force,
just as a certain amount of capital in the bank will
yield a specified sum of interest in a given period
of time. If more than the available interest is with-
drawn, the capital in the bank will be decreased and
gradually exhaust itself completely.

Similarly, if we spend more than our daily allow-
ance of vital force, "Nervous Bankruptcy," that is,
nervous prostration or neurasthenia can only be the
result.

It is the duty of each individual to regulate the
expenditure or loss of vital force according to his
capabilities and interest. He must, therefore, stop
all leaks and guard himself against its waste.

> *"Spiritual element, the vitality, produces the*
> *motive forces of the entity, whether physical*
> *or spiritual. Spiritual forces being the life,*
> *the reproductive principle. As we have mani-*
> *fested, or illustrated, in the physical body,*
> *in nerve tissue: There becomes that principle*
> *of the nerve action and the nerve in action.*
> *That is, with the expression of some condition*
> *bringing distress in the body, the active*

principle is the spirit. The nerve is the soul, for development." 900-17

"In the soul forces, and its indwelling in man, we find the animation, the spiritual element, the soul that developing element, and contained in the brain, in the nerve, in the centers of the whole system. As to the specific centers, nearer those centers of the sensory system, physically speaking." 900-17

"For, as indicated here, the sensory forces are the connections between mind, spirit and body. These are perceiving--not merely vision but feeling, hearing, speaking, all of these responses as by feeling. One becomes attuned to the vibrations even of a room, a place, and other conditions about an environ, through the same tendencies of being or having such attuned to the infinite or to those things that may be very material." 2946-4

"In the physical forces of the body--these respond so long as there are the precautionary measure kept in the manner which has been indicated. When there is neglect, overindulgence or the disregarding of the warnings, there are those disturbing conditions in which the inclinations have been indicated that become a part of the experience." 257-202

There is a well-defined limit to the running of a watch. When the wound spring has spent its force, the mechanism stops.

So also the living forms of vegetable, animal and human life seem to be "wound up" by nature to run a certain length of time, in accordance with principles governing their growth and their development. Even as the healthiest of animals living in the most congenial surroundings in the freedom of nature they do not much exceed their alloted span of life, nor fall much below their alloted span. As a rule, the longer the period

between birth and maturity, the longer the life span
of the animal.

All of the different families of mammals, when
living in freedom, live closely up to the life period
alloted to them by nature. Man is the only exception.
It is claimed that according to the laws of longevity
his average length of life should be considerably over
one hundred years, while according to the latest life-
insurance statistics, the average is about sixty-nine
years. This shows an immense discrepancy between the
possible and the actual longevity of man.

Even this brief span of life means very little
else than weakness, physical and mental suffering and
degeneracy for the majority of the people. Visiting
physicians of the public schools in our large cities
report that seventy-five percent of all the school
children show defective health in one way or another.

These established facts of a greatly impaired
longevity and universal abnormality of the human race
would of themselves indicate that there is something
radically wrong somewhere in the life habits, and in
the thinking of man, and that there is ample reason
for the holistic health reform movement just recently
being organized into a working association.

When people in general become better acquainted
with the laws underlying prenatal and postnatal child
culture, natural living, and the natural treatment or
the prevention of disease, human beings will approach
much more closely the normal in health, beauty, longevity and strength. And there will then arise a true
aristocracy, not of morbid, venous blue-blood, one
pulsating with the rich red blood of vitality and of
health.

However to reach this ideal of perfect physical,
mental and emotional health, the succeeding generations will have to adhere to the naturalistic ways of
living thereby eliminating any and all human ailments.
It cannot be attained by the present generation on the
whole. The enthusiasts who claim that they can, by
their particular methods, achieve perfect health and
live the full term of human life, are destined to
disappointment. We are so handicapped by the mistakes

of the past that the best which most of us adults can do is to "patch up," to attain a reasonable measure, at best, of fair health, and to approach somewhat to nature's intended allotment of life on this earth.

Wild animals living in freedom retain their full vigor unimpaired almost to the end of life. Hunters report that among the great herds of buffalo, elk and deer, the oldest bucks are still the rulers and do maintain their sovereinty over the younger males of the herd solely by reason of their superior strength and prowess. Premature old age, among human beings, is indicated by the early decay of physical and mental powers, as brought on solely by their violations of nature's laws in almost if not all of the ordinary habits of life.

The freer the inflow of the life force into the organism, the greater the vitality, the more there is of strength, of positive resistance to disease and of rapid recuperative power.

In the Edgar Cayce readings we are told that at the very foundation of the manifestation of life lies the principle of polarity, which expresses itself in the duality and unity of positive and negative affinity. The swaying to and fro of the positive and the negative, the desire to balance incomplete polarity, constitute the very ebb and flow of life. So must man keep his body well-balanced.

"Keep the body-physical, then, well-balanced in those infusions of what? that are energies that are positive and negative forces within the material activity, known or classed as the proper chemical balance in same--the fusion of the activities from the material angle that are acid and alkaline; also the potash and the activities in its forces that become the making of materiality by the activity of mind upon same in its influence in the physical forces of self.

"Hence in these manners may the entity, as a physical being, as a mental being, dwell upon the things that are eternal; that it, too, may

*be kept in a balance such as that thy good may
not be evil-spoken of, that thy evil may not
become so overbalanced as to wreck thine own
self in its influences and its activities in
thy conscious walk among thy fellow man."*

826-11

Disease is a disturbed polarity. Exaggerated,
as positive or negative conditions, whether physical,
mental, moral, or spiritual, manifests dis-ease, each
on their own respective planes of being. Foods, medicines, suggestions, and all of the different other
methods of therapeutic treatments exert on the individual subjected to them either a positive or a negative
influence. It is, therefore, of the greatest importance
that the physicians and every one who wishes to live
and work in harmony with nature's laws should understand this all-important question of magnetic polarity.

Lessened vitality means a lowered, slower and
coarser vibration, and this results in lowered resistance to the accumulation of morbid matter, poisons,
disease taints, germs and parasites. This is what we
designate ordinarily as the negative or the acid condition. Its opposite is the alkaline condition. These
must be kept in balance and is known as the PH factor
or the acid-alkaline balance.

*"Keep the body alkaline! Cold germs do not
live in an alkaline system. They do breed in
any acid or excess of acids of ANY character
left in the system." 1947-4*

*"If an alkalinity is maintained in the system
--especially with lettuce, carrots and celery,
these in the blood supply will maintain such
a condition as to immunize a person." 480-19*

*"The diet should be more body building; that
is, less acid foods and more of the alkaline
reacting...Keep close to the alkaline diets,
using fruits, berries, vegetables particularly that carry iron, silicon, phosphorus, and
the like." 480-19*

From this it is evident that negative conditions may be brought about not only by hyper-refinement of the physical organism, but also by clogging it with waste and morbid matter which interfere with the inflow and distribution of the vital force. It must also become apparent that in such cases the natural methods of eliminative treatment, such as pure food diet, exercise, massage, hydrotherapy, etc., are valuable means of removing these obstructions and promote the inflow and free circulation of the positive electric and magnetic life currents of vitality.

Acidity and alkalinity does undoubtedly play an important part in the generation of electricity and magnetism in the human organism. Every electric cell of a battery contains acid and alkaline elements; thus, the human body is similarly made up of electric cells forming a human battery. The glands of the endocrine system acts as dynamos for the recharging of our own human battery.

It has been claimed that what we call vital force is electricity and magnetism, and that these forces are manufactured in the human body. This, however, is but a partial statement of the truth. It is true that vital force manifests in the body as electricity and magnetism, but the life or vital force itself is not generated in the system for it is of the One Force that is responsible for all of the others.

Life is a primary force; it is the source of all activity animating the universe. From this primary force the other secondary forces are derived, such as electricity, magnetism, nerve, muscle and mind force, plus a host of others.

These secondary forces, derived from the One or Divine source cannot be changed back into vital force in the human organism, just as electricity is independent of the incandescent bulb in which it manifests as light.

"Spirit forces are the animation of all life-giving, life-producing forces in animate or inanimate forces. Spiritual elements become corporeal when we speak of the spiritual body

*in a spiritual entity; then composed of spirit,
soul and the superconscious," 900-17*

Our mental and emotional conditions exert also
a most powerful influence upon the inflow and distribution of vital force. The readings describe most
graphically how fear, worry, anxiety, and all kindred
emotions create in the system destructive vibrations
congealing the tissues, clogging the channels of life,
and paralyzing the vital functions of the body. It
shows how the emotional conditions of irritibility,
impatience, anger, etc., have a heating, corroding
effect upon the tissues of the body.

In like manner, all other destructive emotional
vibrations obstruct the flow and normal distribution
of the life forces in and through the organism. While
on the other hand the constructive emotions of faith,
hope, cheerfulness, happiness, and love exert a very
relaxing, harmonizing influence upon the tissues, the
blood vessels and nerve channels, as well as upon the
endocrine system, thus opening wide the floodgates of
the life forces, and raising the discords of weakness,
disease and discontent to the harmonics of health.

*"Keep and make a balance in self, as indicated.
Not only for that pertaining to the physical
and mental, but that purposefulness for which
the activities may be; and knowing for what
expression there is that purposefulness in
thine own spiritual self." 1094-1*

*"But keep a normal balance, not being an
extremist in any direction--whether in diet,
exercise, spirituality or morality--but in
all let there be a co-ordinant influence. For
every phase of the physical, mental and spiritual life is dependent upon the other. They
are one, as the Father-God is One." 2533-3*

Also:

"It would be well for the body to so conduct, so arrange the activities of the body as to be better balanced as to the mental and the physical attributes of the body. Take more outdoor exercise, that--that brings into play the muscular forces of the body. It isn't that the mental should be numbed, or should be cut off from their operations or their activities --but make for a more evenly, a more perfectly balanced body, physical and mental." 341-31

Therefore:

"Keep the self, then, in a perfect balance in the material, the spiritual, the mental welfare and association before others. Let not thy good be evil spoken of, but practice as ye preach..." 341-63

"In finding self as in relationships to the service it may render to others, through those channels that have been indicated, may the greater material gains come to the entity, as well as the balance between the mental and the spiritual." 1602-1

When we fully realize these facts as so stated above, we shall not stand so much in awe of our material bodies. In the past we have been thinking of the body as a solid and imponderable mass difficult to control and change. This conception left us in a condition of utter helplessness and hopelessness in the presence of weakness and disease.

We now think of the body as composed of minute corpuscles rotating around one another within the atom at relatively immense speeds. We know that in similar manners the atoms vibrate in the molecule, the molecules in the cell, the cells in the organ, and all of the organs in the body; the whole capable of being changed by a change in the vibrations of its particles.

Thus the erstwhile solid physical mass appears plastic and fluidic, readily swayed and changed by

the vibratory harmonies or discords of thoughts and
emotions as well as by foods, medicines and therapeutic
treatments.

Under the old conception the mind fell readily
under the control of the body and became the abject
slave of its physical conditions, swayed by fear and
apprehension under every sensation of physical weakness, discomfort or pain. The servants lorded it with
a high hand over the master of the house, and the
result was chaos. Under the new conception, control
is placed where it belongs. It is assumed by the real
master of the house, the soul-man, and the servants,
the physical members of the body, remain obedient to
his bidding.

This is the new man, the ideal progeny of New
Thought and Higher Philosophy. Understanding the body
structure, the laws of its being, and the operation of
the life elements within it, the super-man retains
perfect poise and confidence under the most trying
circumstances. Animated by an abounding faith in the
supremacy of the vital healing forces within him and
sustained by the power of his sovereign will, he
governs his body as perfectly as the artist controls
his violin, and attunes its vibrations to nature's
harmonies of health and happiness.

Thus:

*"To live--to be--and to maintain bodily acti-
vity unto the glory of the Creative Forces--
is the purpose of the entrance of each entity
into material consciousness."* 2981-1

CHAPTER TWELVE

PERIODICITY: THE LAW OF SEVENS

In many forms of acute disease, "crises" develop with marked regularity and in well defined periodicity. This phenomena has been observed and described by many physicians.

It is not so well known, however, that in the cure of chronic diseases also, crises do develop in accordance with certain laws of periodicity.

Periodicity is governed by the spiritual law or the Law of Sevens, which seems to be the basic law governing the vibratory activities of the planetary universe.

The harmonics of heat, light, sound, electricity, magnetism, and atomic structure and arrangement run in scales of seven.

"Seven signify the spiritual forces, as are seen in all the ritualistic order of any nature; as seen in the dividing up of conditions, whether they be of the forces of nature or those that react to the sensual forces of man in any character." 5751-1

The law of sevens govern the days of the week, the phases of the moon, and the menstrual periods of the woman. Every observing physician is aware of its influence on feverish, nervous and psychic diseases.

The law of sevens dominates the life of nations, of individuals, and of everything that lives and has periods of birth, growth, fruitage and declination.

"The whole anatomical structure is changed in each cycle--or every seven years." 3236-1

"For the body renews itself, every atom, in seven years.

*"How have ye lived for the last seven years?
and then the seven years before? what would
ye do with thy mind and thy body if they were
wholly restored to normalcy in this experience?
Would these be put to the use of gratifying
thine own appetites as at first? Will these be
used for the magnifying of the appreciation
of love toward the infinite? 3684-1*

*"As is understood by some, thought by many,
there is within each physical being the elements whereby the organs and their activities
and functionings are enabled within themselves
to supply that needed for replenishing or
rebuilding their own selves.*
*"This may be done, as comprehended, in a period
of every seven years. Thus it is a slow process, but it is a growth in the energies of
the body-force itself. For it is either from
potash, iodine, soda or fats, that each of
these in their various combinations and mul-
titude activities supply all the other forces
of the body energies. Yet in each body there
is born or projected that something of the
soul-self also." 3124-1*

Over two thousand years ago Pythagoras and Hippocrates distinctly recognized and proclaimed the Law of
Crises in its bearing on the cure of chronic diseases.
They taught that alternating, well-defined periods of
improvement and of crises were determined and governed
by the law of periodicity and the law of numbers (the
Septimal Law).

The following quotations are taken from the Ency-
clopedia Britannica, Vol. XV, p. 800:

"But this artistic completeness was closely connected with the 'third cardinal virtue' of Hippocratic
medicine--the clear recognition of disease as being
equally with life a process governed by what we should
now call natural laws, which could be known by observation and which indicated the spontaneous and normal
direction of recovery, by following which alone could

the physician succeed...

"Another Hippocratic doctrine, the influence of which is not even yet exhausted, is that of the healing power of nature. Not that Hippocrates taught, as he was afterwards reproached with teaching, that nature is sufficient for the cure of diseases; for he held strongly the efficacy of art. But he recognized, at least in acute diseases, a natural process which the humours went through--being first of all *crude*, then passing through coction or digestion, and finally being expelled by resolution or *crisis* through one of the natural channels of the body. The duty of physicians was to foresee these changes, 'to assist or not to hinder them,' so that 'the sick man might conquer the disease with the help of the physician.' The times at which crises were to be expected were naturally looked for with anxiety; and it was a cardinal point in the Hippocrates system to foretell them with precision. Hippocrates, influenced as is thought by the Pythagorean doctrine of numbers, taught that they were to be expected on days fixed by certain numerical rules, in some cases on odd, in others on even numbers--the celebrated doctrine of 'critical days!' It follows from what has been said that *prognosis,* or the art of foretelling the course and event of the disease, was a strong point with the Hippocratic physicians. In this perhaps they have never been excelled. Diagnosis, or the recognition of the disease, must have been necessarily imperfect, when no scientific nosology, or system of disease existed, and the knowledge of anatomy was quite inadequate to allow of a precise determination of the seat of disease; but symptoms were no doubt observed and interpreted skillfully. The pulse is not spoken of in any of the works now attributed to Hippocrates himself, though it is mentioned in other works of the collection.

"In the treatment of diseases, the Hippocrates school attached great importance to diet, the variation necessary in different diseases being minutely defined. ...In chronic cases, diet, exercise and other natural methods were chiefly relied upon."

These wonderful truths, with other wisdom of the

ancients were lost in the spiritual darkness of the
Middle Ages. Modern medicine looks upon those claims
and teachings of the Hippocratic school as "super-
tition without any foundation in fact." However the
great sages of antiquity, drawing upon a source of
ancient wisdom, deeply hidden from the self-satisfied
scribes and wise men of the schools, have after all
proclaimed the truth.

Every case of chronic disease properly treated
by natural methods proves the reality and stability
of the law of crises. It is, therefore, a standing
wonder and surprise to one "who knows," that this all
important and self-evident law is practically unknown
to the disciples of the regular schools of medicine.
And in the words of Edgar Cayce:

> *"In this present experience, these of study
> --these of the stars--these of mystic numbers,
> places, conditions, are all absorbing to the
> entity. Rather apply same as to the relation-
> ships of numbers, mystic forces and symbols
> to that of the creative energies as are given
> through Him that came as the ransom for many
> making man one with the Creative Energy in the
> life, in the manner of showing forth to others
> that the pathway may be led in the direction
> where all may be one with that Energy. So, in
> numbers--so, in mystic forces--so, in the cycle
> of things--may this entity, applying same with
> the life as led by the Master, guide many--as
> aids in physical, in material, in spiritual
> life." 256-1*

> *"Q.- What is meant by the cycle of things?
> "A.- That to which an attunement turns in its
> orbit about an influence; for, as is seen, in
> any cycle--cycle means...in the beginning is
> the end; for when there is the beginning it
> means only a change. A cycle is the change,
> or the using up of the force, energy to where
> the change may be definitely set as change.
> That is a cycle, whether of the life in a*

*manifested form--in body, in mind, in stars,
in the whole of ANY--as a change, a cycle."*
256-2

So:

*"Remember, the body rebuilds and replenishes
itself continually. What portion would be the
more active in its changes than those that
are the channels for these very changes--the
digestive forces of the body; the lungs, the
liver, the heart, the digestive system, the
pancreas, the spleen? All of these change the
more often, so that when it is ordinarily
termed that the body has changed each atom in
seven years, these organs have changed almost
seven times during those seven years!*
*"Hence these should not disturb the body,
provided the proper balances are being kept
in the system." 796-2*

In accordance with the law of periodicity, the
SIXTH period in any cycle of seven periods is marked
by reactions, changes, revolutions, or "crises," It
is, therefore, looked upon by popular intuition as an
"unlucky" period. Friday, the sixth day of the week,
is regarded as an unlucky day; Friday is "hangman's
day"; according to tradition the Master, Jesus, was
crucified on a Friday.

Counting from the sixth or "Friday" period in any
given number of hours, days, weeks, months, years, or
groups of years, as the case may be, every succeeding
seventh period is characterized by crises.

This explains why 13 is considered an "unlucky"
number. It represents the second critical or "Friday"
period.

However, there is really no cause for this super-
titious fear of Friday and the number 13. But this is
due to a lack of understanding of nature's laws. By
intelligent cooperation with these laws we may turn
the critical periods in our lives into "healing crises"
and beneficial changes.

We should never fear the crises periods of the

larger life and the changes occurring in our outward
circumstances which they may bring, any more than we
should fear crises in the physical body.

A thorough understanding of the nature and purpose
of "healing crises" in acute and chronic diseases has
taught me the nature and purpose of "evil" in general.
It has made me understand more clearly the meaning
of "Resist not Evil" and the saying: "We are punished
by our sins, not for our sins." It has shown me that
evil is not a punishment or a curse, but a necessary
complement of good; that it is corrective and educational in its purposes; that it remains with us only
as long as we need its salutary lessons.

The evil of any physical disease is not due to
accident or to the arbitrary rulings of a capricious
Providence, nor is it always "error of mortal mind."
From the Cayce philosophy and its practical application
I have learned that, barring accidents and conditions
and surroundings unfavorable to human life, or that
the works of God may be manifest, it is caused in most
every instance by violations of the physical, mental
and spiritual laws of our being. So the social, political and industrial evil of the larger life is
brought about by violations of the same laws in the
respective domains of that life and its resulting
actions and reactions.

So long as there are transgression of the laws
of our being resulting in hereditary and in acquired
disease encumbrances, we must expect reactions which
may become either disease crises or healing crises.
Likewise, so long as ignorance, selfishness, and self-
indulgence continue to create evil in other domains
of life, we must, therefore, expect also the occurrence
of crises, of action and reaction, of harmony and
revolution. When knowledge, self-control and altruism
become the sole motives of our actions, evil and the
crises it necessitates will naturally disappear.

*"The motivative forces in life itself are the
composite activity of the spirit of life,
hence, as individuals first, we recognize that
each activity, each expression of self in its*

relationships to that from, without and that
from within, is the expression of that we have
done about--or with--the knowledge and the
consciousness of His presence abiding with
each." 262-31

Therefore, we should not be afraid of changes and crises periods but learn to co-operate with them clear-eyed and strong-willed. Thus they will result in our improvement and further the growth and development of our being.

Life is growth and growth is change. The only death is stagnation. The loss of children, friends, home, and fortune may seem for the time being as an overwhelming calamity; but if met in the right spirit, such losses will prove as stepping-stones to greater opportunities and higher achievements. Of this, I speak with conviction for I have gone through it personally myself.

Many people formerly looked upon their disease condition as a great misfortune and an undeserved punishment. And such harships has brought so many of them to the awareness of a higher philosophy as contained in the Cayce readings, or similar teachings, showing the necessity for complying with the natural laws of being. They now look upon the former evil as the greatest blessing in their lives, because it has taught them how to become the masters of their own destiny instead of remaining as the plaything of the destructive forces of nature.

"First there is the Destiny, as we have indi-
cated, of the Mind; that is both material and
spiritual.
"Then there is the Destiny of the Body, as we
have indicated. And it is held by some, that
the body being of the earth-earthy it is born
into the earth, dies and returns to earth.
This has been set by the sages of old, and
would indicate that the body--being of that
phase of experience or existence--remains in
its sphere; that while changes come about, it
remaineth." 262-86

Why should we fear even the greatest of all crises, "physical death," when it, also, is only the gateway to a larger life, greater opportunities, and more beautiful surroundings? Why should we mourn and grieve over the death of friends and relatives, when they have only emigrated to another, better country?

Suppose we ourselves had to enter upon the great journey today or tomorrow, would we not be glad to meet some of our relatives on the other side, and to be welcomed, advised, and guided by them, in the new surroundings?

Therefore we should not fear, nor endeavor to avoid the crises in any and all domains of life and action, but meet them and co-operate with them fearlessly and intelligently. They then will always make for greater opportunity and higher accomplishment.

"There should not be the attempt upon the part of any in the material activities to make for distresses about the body. For these changes that come in the experience of the soul and spiritual activity of a body are the natural consequences. And these should be viewed from that ideal; that those forces which make for the greater construction should be kept in the spiritual manner for the body." 1059-1

CHAPTER THIRTEEN

LAW OF SEVENS: APPLIED INDIVIDUALLY

Applied to the life of the individual, the law of periodicity manifests itself as follows:

Human life on the earth-plane is divided into periods of seven years. The first seven years represent the period of infancy. With the next seven, the years of childhood, begins individual responsibility, the conscious discernment between right and wrong. The third group comprises the years of adolescence; the fourth marks the attainment of full growth. Nearly all civilized countries take cognizance of this by fixing the legal age at 21.

The 28th year, the beginning of the fifth period, is another milestone along the road to development.

The sixth period, beginning at the age of thirty-five and ending at forty-two, is marked by reactions, changes, and crises. It may, therefore, seem to be an "unlucky period; but if we understand the law, and learn to comply with it, we shall then be better and stronger in every way after we have passed over this trying period.

During the seventh period, the effects of the sixth or "Crises" period continues to adjust itself. It is a period of reconstruction, of recuperation and rest, and thus is the best preparation for a new cycle of sevens which begins with the fiftieth year.

"Individuals in the earth move from cycle to cycle in their own development, in their relationships with individuals and with the activities having to do with that which may be accomplished in meeting certain conditions."
993-4
"Each cycle brings a soul entity to another crossroad, or another urge from one or several of its activities in the material plane." 3128-1

In this connection it is interesting to note that the Mosaic law recognized the law of periodicity, and fixed upon Sunday as the first day or "birthday" of the week, and upon Saturday (the Sabbath) as the last or "rest" day, in which to prepare for another period of seven days.

Orthodox science now admits that the normal length of human life should be about one hundred and fifty years. This would constitute three cycles of forty-nine years each, the first corresponding to the youthful cycle, the second to the cycle of maturity, and the third or last cycle to that of fruition.

However, the Cayce readings have the following to say on longevity:

> "For as the body is the storehouse of all influences and forces from without, it has the abilities for the creating--with the correct firing or fuel for the body--that which is able to sustain, not only sustain but to recuperate and to rebuild, revitalize, regenerate the activities of the body." 1334-1

> "Q.- May I expect to have a long life...?
> "A.- It's well to expect it, even though it may be cut short! But these again depend upon the activities of the entity. If there are the setting of the purposes in the experience of the entity that life is to be, the life is an expression of the Creative Forces, the results are long life." 1233-1

> "For life itself--as has been given--is a manifestation of God. Thus a soul, an entity, may hold on to life so long as it wills to obey that which is the consciousness as to the relationship of the entity to life--or God." 2390-2

Civilization has largely stood for artificiality of life and for artificial gambits. A higher civilization, yet to come, will combine today's most exquisite culture of heart and mind and soul with true simplicity and naturalness of living. Excessive meat-eating, strong spices and condiments, alcohol, coffee, tea, overwork, nightwork, fear, worry, sensuality, foul air, improper breathing, lack of exercise, all of these and the many other evils of an hyper-civilization, have also contributed their share in the creating of universal degeneracy on the civilized nations of earth.

When the unnatural habits of life just alluded to, have lowered the vitality and favored the accumulation of waste matter and poisons to such an extent that the sluggish bowels, kidneys, skin, and the other organs of elimination are unable to keep a clean house, nature has to resort to other, and sometimes to more radical means of purification, else we would choke in our own impurities. These forcible house-cleansings of nature are colds, catarrhs, skin eruptions, boils, diarrhea, ulcers, abnormal perspiration, hemorrages, and the many other forms of similar diseases. All of these negative manifestations are thereby urging us to prescribe changes of old habits into new and more positive ones.

> *"In the gratifying of a desire, these become habit-forming; in the manner of the effect then of the drug and the effects of alcohol upon the system weakening the will and thus weakening the coordination between the manifestation of spiritual truth with material gratification of flesh desires.*
> *"Then, WE would give that not only must the body-mind turn to the spiritual promises that are a part of its mental and spiritual self, but the environment must be changed; so that the spiritual promises may be put to active service and work to replace the habits of doing GOOD, doing right, doing justice, being merciful."* 1427-1

> *"For what one builds in the subconscious of itself, it becomes—rather as a habit, like any form of activity by the voluntary motions of the body-forces."* 3287-2

"For just as habits and appetites for activities in association with others become a part of the mental and the reactions in the sensitive forces of the nervous system, so are they builded to become a part of the whole experience--and must be met within self sooner or later." 1691-1

Therefore:

"That brings often the ability to attune self through that as of the habit; for, as has been given, the physical is of the material. The mental or habit forming is of the subconscious, and oft through the subconscious only may the superconsciousness be brought into being. Control the habit, and let not the habit control self." 137-127

However:

"For the body has been accustomed to limp and it'll keep on limping until it breaks itself of the habit, by forming other habits. We break a habit by forming a habit. This we all do. So does this body. Think constructively. Be constructive but do keep up those suggestions we have indicated if we would eliminate these disturbances from the body." 3287-2

"In the present when evil has taken hold it forms itself into those influences which are called habits, or inclinations, or intents; and it is necessary to eliminate these from the purposes and aims and desires of individuals." 281-41

Yet:

"...each soul, each mind, each entity is endowed with its choice. And the choice is the result of the application of self in

relationships to that which is its ideal--and finds manifestation in what individuals call habit, or subconscious activity. Yet it has its inception in that of choice." 830-2

Under the influences of wrong habits of living and the suppressive treatment of disease, all forms of waste and morbid matter affect the cells, and obstruct the tiny spaces between them. This is bound to interfere with the normal functions of the organism, and in time will lead to deterioration and organic destruction.

Every individual cell must be supplied with food and oxygen. These it receives from the red arterial blood. The cells must also be provided with an outlet for their waste products. This is furnished by the venous circulation, which represents the drainage system of the body. If this drainage is defective the effects upon the organism is similar to the effects produced upon a house when the excretions and discharges of its inhabitants are allowed to remain in it, and vermins are entertained.

Furthermore, every cell must be in unobstructed communication with the nerve currents of the organism. But most important of all, it must in itself, be in touch with the sympathetic nervous system and, it in turn with the endocrine system, through which it receives the impulses of the Life Force. It not only vivifies and controls all involuntary functions of the cells and organs in the human body, but, it is also the mysterious connecting or staging areas for the interaction of the physical, the mental and the spiritual planes of being.

The Cayce readings state the following:

"First, this shows that there is innate in each physical individual that channel through which the psychic or the spiritual forces, that are manifest in a material world, may function. They are known as glands, and affect the organs of the system." 294-141

"But there are physical contacts which the

anatomist finds not, or those who would look
for imaginations of the minds. Yet it is found
that within the body there are channels, there
are ducts, there are glands, there are acti-
vities that performs no one knows what! in a
living, moving thinking being. In many indi-
viduals such become dormant, many have become
atrophied. Why? Non-usage, non-activity! Be-
cause only the desires of the appetites, self-
indulgences and such, have so glossed over or
used up the abilities in these directions that
they become only wastes as it were in the
spiritual life of an individual who has so
abused or misused those abilities that have
been given him for the greatest activity."
                                    281-41

"Then we find the endocrine system—not glands
but system—is that which is disseminated
throughout the whole of the body, as related
to the physical forces of same, and may be
studied or may be followed in their relation-
ship not only to the physical structural forces
of the body but to what we call hereditary and
environmental forces and how they may be
expected to react upon the system." 281-38

In many ways we find proof of the fact that there
are some interesting results caused by some mysterious
power that seems to be different from anything mechanical, electrical, mental or physical, and therefore
must evidently be a force that is not as yet explain-
able scientifically.

When we recall how many centuries electricity has
been known, used and investigated, while even today
it cannot be said that it is understood satisfactorily.
We may feel more reconciled as to the comparative
ignorance that exists regarding this force, though it
has been used and studied on and off for ages by those
suspect of its existence. It is more or less consciously felt at one time or another by most every one,
and we see here a strong possibility that marvelous
development, and application of this force may, at

times, reward the successful user.

In our natural haste to satisfy curiosity we must not forget that even the highest of science can never explain the phenomena of nature herself. It can only discover results, classify them and deduce a theory to link them logically together; but these hypotheses are not true explanations by any means.

This desire for an "understanding" of every new phenomena has ever hindered the practical employment of this force for the serious concerns of daily life. It has been relegated to the deceivers, until it is popularly identified with hallucinations and humbug. To rescue this valuable endowment of nature from the unwarranted neglect which it has suffered, because of ill-advised prejudice, has been the underlying purpose of these chapters with their accompanying explanations. Let us then impartially consider some of the statements from the readings of Cayce which are based upon and a widespread region of homogeneous facts, especially in relationship to that as related in oriental literature and the Bible's Book of Revelation. The term used in the readings is "Kundaline," an Hindu term representing this life force.

> *"As for the physical forces, the weakness in the nerve tensions through the body has come from periods when there has been the opening of centers of the body without direction to the use of the energies that have been and are created in and through the kundaline forces as they act along the spine."* 5286-1

> *"...the third cervical...the 9th dorsal and ...the 4th lumbar...*
> *"These are the three centers through which there is the activity of the kundaline forces that act as suggestions to the spiritual forces for distribution through the seven centers of the body."* 3676-1

Therefore:

*"As the body-mind entertains and enters into
the raising of the kundaline influence through
the body, surround self with the light of the
Christ Consciousness--by thought, by word of
mouth, by impressing it upon self. And in that
light there may be never any harm to self or
to the emotions of the body, or any fear of
the mental and spiritual self being entertained
or used by the dark influence."* 2329-3

Hence:

*"How many dispositions have you seen in the
body? These are all activities of the kundaline
forces acting upon some reactory force in the
centers of the body. These are well to be
controlled, or maintained, but purposely--not
for selfish motives; to be sure, individual,
but creative."* 1861-11

*"For, when this has arisen--and is disseminated
properly through the seven centers of the
body, it has purified the body from all desire
of sex relationships."* 2329-1

There is some force, means, or agent by which mind
is enabled to act on matter, and yet which is itself
entirely distinct from mind or matter.

This agent must be ranked with the other kindred
attractive forces of nature, such as electricity,
gravity, capillarity and adhesion. It is quite similar
in its operation to electricity and magnetism, and
perhaps is invariably accompanied by them.

The process of initiation into the mysteries of
a reality in connection with miraculous feats, led
all the ancient philosophers to attempt a solution and
understanding of this force. Galen said, "These things
I have not tested, neither have I denied them because,
if we had not seen the magnet attracting iron, we would
not believe it." Cicero, in like scientific manner
said, "I am contented in that even if I am ignorant,
yet what does happen I know." And different minds,

have come to substantiate the very same conclusions.

Various terms have been applied to this mysterious force. Plato called it the "soul of the world." Others called it the "plastic spirit of the world," while Descartes gave it the afterward popular name of "animal spirits." The stoics called it simply "nature," which is now changed generally to "nervous principle." However, the Cayce readings term it the "kundaline" after the oriental name for this force.

In the earliest days there prevailed a theory that all motive influences in nature--which we know to be, as they insisted, intermediate between spirit and matter--make up the soul of the world, and which embraces all human spirits. Long before Plato, it was believed that there is one great pervading, embracing, universal spirit, filling immensity. This was the power motivating all material things.

Cicero, in commenting on this theory, says: "In what way is this mysterious influence communicated, can be no more explained than can any other mysteries of nature's simplest operations, as for example, the growth of plants.

Various have been the philosophies and theologies that this primal hypotheses has been made trying to establish it as fact. This, however, need not blind us to the theory itself, so far as it relates to phenomena that seems to occur in accord with it. But, two centuries since, an eminent astronomer, Huygens, whose researches perfected the pendulum and the air pump, adopted a corresponding theory, and called it, the all-pervading substance, "Ether." In this he was joined by other mathematicians and this view is now generally accepted today.

We may therefore feel very confident that there is, what we might call a universal atmosphere which encompasses, at least, all beings on this globe. Just as we individually breathe the same air and take our separate lives from its chemicals, so this ethereal principle sustain our power of activity and personal influence, and is everywhere ready to be judiciously used, or refused, as we would choose.

Physiologists had long entertained the general

conception of some subtle fluid, spirit, or influence
manifesting from the brain to the muscles, along the
sympathetic nervous system. This will probably never
be fully explained, but the principle once established
does specify that there does exist in the animal or
human economy a power of determining the development
of electrical excitement capable of being transmitted
along the nerves and unknown channels. It becomes then
an easy step to refer, therefore, to the origin of the
seven spiritual centers of the body and their activities, to the more fully detailed descriptions given
in the Edgar Cayce readings.

> *"There are centers in a physical body through
> which all phases of the entity's being coor-
> dinated with one another; as in the physical
> functioning there are the pulsations, the heart
> beat, the lungs, the liver, and all the organs
> of the body. They each have a function to per-
> form. They each are dependent upon the other
> yet they function according to those directions
> of the mental self--or the nervous systems.*
> *"Yet while the brain and the cords through
> which the nerve function are the channels,
> these are not the mental consciousness, though
> it is through the nerve plasm that the nervous
> systems carry impulses to the various forces
> of the system." 2114-1*

> *"Then, there are centers, areas, conditions,
> in which there evidently must be that contact
> between the physical, the mental and the spi-
> ritual.*
> *"The spiritual contact is through the glandular
> forces of creative energies; not encased only
> within the (Leydig) lyden gland of reproduc-
> tion, for this is ever--so long as life exists
> --in contact with the brain cells through
> which there is the constant reaction through
> the pineal.*
> *"Hence we find these become subject not only
> to the intent and purpose of the individual*

*entity or soul upon the entrance, but are
constantly under the influences of all the
centers of the mind and the body through which
the impulse pass in finding a means or manner
of expression in the mental or brain itself.
"Thus we find the connection, the association
of the spiritual being with the mental self,
at those centers from which the reflexes react
to all of the organs, all of the emotions, all
of the activities of a physical body." 263-13*

However:

*"AS hath been indicated for the group, for
members of same, there is that line, that
connection , that point of CONTACT in the body-
physical to the spiritual forces as manifest
through same. There are centers of the body
through which contacts are made, or are physically active, that at times, at all times,
produce a sound. It may not be heard, it may
not be always experienced by the individual,
but finds expression in emotions of varied
centers, varied characters." 281-27*

*"The seven centers of the body--where sympa-
thetic and cerebro-spinal coordinate the more;
1st, 2nd and 3rd cervical; 1st and 2nd dorsal;
5th and 6th dorsal; 9th dorsal; 11th and 12th
dorsal, and through the lumbar and sacral
areas. These are the sources. This is not an
infection--it is the lack of coordination
between the impulses of the mental self and
the central nerve and blood supply." 3428-1*

*"There are certain centers along the spine
where there is greater coordination between
the central nervous system and the sympathetic
and those of the organs of sensory forces. So,
as we would find, first, we would, through
hydrotherapy, thoroughly purify the bodily
forces. Three to six, then, thorough fume*

baths; then thorough massages, including
colonic baths. Do these at Reilly's. Thus we
will purify the body by removing a great deal
of dross that is preventing better conditions."
                                        5401-1
For:

"If ye will study to UNDERSTAND the opening
of the channels or the centers for the deeper
meditation, then the spiritual and psychic
awakening may be brought forth. But do not
allow self to be overcome with this until ye
understand how and why centers are opened in
meditation. This is a psychic experience."
                                        1552-1
"There are those definite centers from which
impulses arise; as the body has experienced
and does experience through meditation, or
prayer, or vibratory forces being aroused from
the centers of the bodily force as they connect
with the sensory system as related to the
cerebro-spinal." 1770-1

Therefore:

"Do not attempt to open any of the centers of
the book until self has been tried in the
balance of self's own conscious relationship
to the Creative Forces and not found wanting
by the spiritual answer in self to that rather
as is seen in the manner in which the book
itself becomes as that in the whole body which
may be assimilated by the body, when taken
properly. In these then there has been set as
ye have in thine outline. These are well. Do
do not misuse them." 281-29

"And here we find some of those conditions of
which many bodies should be warned--the opening
of the centers in the body-spiritual without
correctly directing same, which may oft lead
to wrecking of the body-physical and sometimes
mental.

"Know where you are going before you start out, in analyzing spiritual and mental and material things." 3428-1

Also:

"There has long been sought, by a few, the interpretation of the seven centers; and many have in various stages of awareness, or development, placed the association or connection between physical, mental and spiritual in varied portions of the body. Some have interpreted as of the mind, motivated by impulse; and thus called the center from which the mind acts.
"This is only relatively so, as will be understood by those who analyze those conditions presented through these interpretations; for in fact the body, the mind and soul are ONE, in the material manifestation. Yet in analyzing them, as given through the Revelation of John, they are active in the various influences that are a part of each living organism conceived in the forces making up that known as man; that power able to conceive--in mind--of God, and to demonstrate same in relationships to others; that in mind able to conceive of manners for the destruction of its fellow man, little realizing that it is self being destroyed by that very activity!" 281-51

And the Revelation:

"In the material world, in the anatomy books that have been written by some, attempted by many, there is considered only the physical channel, and not the mental and spiritual attributes and activities. But if ye are studying these (activities of the glands in the light that they are to be applied in the interpreting of Revelation, then the mental and spiritual must also be taken into consiration." 281-49

*"And then the Revelation; knowing this--the
Revelation--is a description of, a possibility
of thy own consciousness; and not as a histo-
rical fact, not as a fancy, but as that thy own
soul has sought throughout its experiences
through the phases of thy abilities,   the
faculties of thy mind and body, the emotions
of all thy complex--as it may appear--system."*
                                    1473-1

*"In giving the interpretation of this parti-
cular portion of the Revelation, it must be
kept in mind that, as has been indicated, while
many of the references--or all--refer to the
physical body as the pattern, there is that
as may be said to be the literal and the
spiritual and the metaphysical interpretation
of almost all portions of the Scripture, and
especially of the Revelation as given by John.
"Yet all of these to be true, to be practical,
to be applicable in the experiences of individuals, must coordinate; or be as one, even
as the Father, the Son and the Holy Spirit!*
                                    281-31

The above opens up an immeasurable field for the
imagination, and satisfies us in the fact that we are
all the more closely linked with the universe and its
wonderful secrets and potent forms, than would seem
possible to the casual thinkers. We would wish that
this information might act as an inspiration to the
readers of this book, urging them steadily on through
the necessary study for understanding and applying
that, that will prepare them to lay hold upon with an
almost herculean grasp of the powers that a lavisly,
beneficient nature has provided for our use.

Humanity is hemmed in by so many varied influences
that, from time immemorial, no real effort has been
made to gain control of the impulses that run rampant
in the universe. It has been, and still is easier to
let things go as they will rather than exert the will
to direct them constructively.

All of us are creatures of emotions, passions,
circumstances and accident. What the mind will be,

what the heart will be, what the body will be, are problems that are shaped to the drift of life, even when special attention is given to any of them.

If you will sit down and think awhile, and you will be surprised to know how much of your life has been mere drift; how little you have done toward the finding out of the power that operates in the human organism, whence it came, how it is lost, misused and how it may be utilized to the best advantage.

Look at any created life, and see how strong are the efforts to express itself. The tree shoots its branches toward the sunlight; struggles through its leaves to inhale the oxygen; and, even underground, sends forth its roots in search of water and nutrients. This you call inanimate life; but this represents the force that comes from some source of power having an intelligence able to keep all things in equilibrium.

Man is a higher animal, and animal life is but a higher vegetation. There are more millions of flesh cells in your body than your mind could conceive or your pencil could write in figures, yet not one of these cells originate otherwise than in a vegetable. Nor could it have originated but for some force that existed in and of the cell itself.

There is no place on this globe where energy is not found. The air is so loaded with it, that in the cold north the sky shines in boreal rays; and wherever the frigid temperature yields to the warm air so the electrical conditions alarms man. Water (H_2O) is but a liquid union of gases, and is charged with electrical, mechanical and chemical energies, any one of which is capable of doing great service or great damage to man. Even ice, as water in its coldest phase, has energy, for it is not subdued, nor even stilled; its force has the capacity for breaking mountain rocks into small fragments.

This energy about us, we drink in from water, eat in from the food and breathe in from the air. Not one chemical molecule is ever free from it; nor can atoms exist without it. We are a combination of individual energies but yet of a single energy, power or force. It is from one universal source.

"*All force is as one force. Hence the universal forces. All knowledge is as one knowledge; hence may be attained from the universal force or knowledge.*" 254-30

"*It will be found that all have their place; for, as we have given, every force--in its manifestation--is from the One, or God. And that which is manifested in material things is a result, and not the motive force; for mind, mental, (which may not be seen with the spiritual eye) is the builder.*" 347-2

"*Know first that the knowledge of God is a growing thing, for ye grow in grace, in knowledge, in understanding as ye apply that YE KNOW. But remember, as has been given by Him, to know to do good and do it not is sin.*
"*In the interpretation then of the Revelation as given by John in Patmos: This was John's Revelation of his experience, and interpreted in the individual by the application of the body of self as a pattern with the attributes physically, mentally, spiritually, in their respective spheres for thine own revelation.*
"*For this to be practical, to be applicable in the experience of each soul, it must be an individual experience; and the varied experiences or activities of an entity in its relationship to the study of self, are planned, builded, workable in the pattern as John has given in the Revelation.*
"*Each attribute of the body, whether organ or functioning or the expression of same, becomes then in the experience of each soul as a seeker first. Seek and ye shall find, knock and it shall be opened unto you!*
"*Then in thy study, for those who would become Glad Helpers, in the physical, in the moral, in the mental, in the spiritual life of each soul: Condemn no one. Love all. Do good. And ye may experience it all.*" 281-30

CHAPTER FOURTEEN

TWOFOLD ATTITUDE OF BODY, MIND AND SOUL

There is nothing contradictory or incompatible in the teachings of the natural healing philosophies concerning the physical and meta-physical methods of treating human ailments. Both the independent and the dependent attitudes of body, mind and soul are both good and true, and may be entertained as one and at the same time. It is necessary for us to rely on our own personal efforts in carrying out the dictates of reason and of commons sense. But this need not prevent us from praying for and confidently expecting larger inflows of vital power and intuitional discernment from the source of all intelligence and power in the innermost parts of our being.

This two-fold attitude of body, mind and soul is justified not only by reason and intuition, but also by the anatomical structure of the human organism and its physiological and psychological faculties, capaties and powers.

"For, ye find thyself body, mind, soul. These three bear witness in the earth. And the Christ Consciousness, the Holy Spirit AND thy guardian angel bear witness in the spirit." 2246-1

"In the body, then, we have the body, the mind, the soul; each representing a phase of man's experience or consciousness." 262-86

"The body, the mind, the soul are one within the physical forces; for the body is indeed the temple of the living God. In each entity there is that portion which is a part of the universal force, and is that which lives on. All must coordinate and cooperate." 1593-1

145

*"For while the body, the mind, the soul may
be spoken of as three divisions of the one, it
is only the conception of their oneness--as
it relates to the Oneness without--that the
strength of the abilities is aroused to fulfill
the purpose for which ye entered this experience."* 1580-1

Therefore:

*"Man finds himself a body, a mind, a soul. The
body is self-evident. The mind also is at times
understood. The soul or the spiritual portion
is hoped for, and one may only discern same
from a spiritual consciousness.*
*"The body, mind and soul are as the Father, the
Son and the Holy Spirit--just as infinity in
its expression to the finite mind is expressed
in time, space and patience."* 2879-1

*"We three are one, even as the Father, the Son,
and the Holy Ghost. As we abide in thee, and
through the various elements, the various
attributes of each, they manifest in and
through the various forces of bodies in thee."*
137-127

The activities of the human organism are governed
by two different systems of nerves, the sympathetic
and the cerebro-spinal. However, the sympathetic nervous system along with the endocrine system is that
conveyor of vital force from the mind and soul elements
to the organs and the cells of the body. Just what this
vital force is and where it ultimately comes from, we
do not know. It is a manifestation of that force we
call God, Nature, Life, the Higher Power, or Divine
Law within and without.

*"For thy Father-God is within self and without.
Then as ye treat thy fellow man, ye are
treating thy Maker. These are immutable,
unchangeable laws of divine origin--not man's
concept."* 3198-3

"Hence they partook of, and became a portion of, absorbing all WITHIN themselves so that every element WITHOUT a human body is--or finds an expression--within some form, or some activity of a living organism. Hence the various activities as are manifested without find a response within the physical organism."

262-19

The more we study the anatomy, physiology and psychology of the human organism, the more we wonder at its marvelous complexity and ingenuity of structure and function of forces acting within and without. In every existing moment of life there are enacted in our bodies innumerable mechanical, chemical, and psychological miracles. Who, or what, performs these miracles? We do not know. Yet every moment of our lives depends upon the infinite care and wisdom of this unknown, impersonal, twofold aspect of Divine intelligence and power, entitled Lord God in the Good Book.

Why, then, should we not trust One so faithful? Why should we not ask aid from One so powerful? And why should we not seek enlightenment from One so wise and so benevolent?

However, not all of the human entity is entirely dependent upon such an intelligent impersonal power, or are all its functions independently involuntary. Within the house prepared by the Divine Intelligence, there dwells a sovereign in his own right and by his own might. He is endowed with freedom of desire, of choice, and of action. He creates in his brain the nerve power which control the voluntary activities of the body, and from these brain centers he sends his commands through the fibers of the motor nerves to the voluntary muscles and makes them do his bidding; some he commands to walk, others to laugh, to eat, etc.

This independent principle in man we call the ego, the personal or individual intelligence. It imagines, desires, reasons, plans, and works out, by the power of free will and independent choice, its own salvation or destruction, physically, mentally, morally, and spiritually. By means of the motor nervous system, this thinker and doer directs and controls from his headquarters in the brain all the voluntary functions, capacities, and powers of the human organism.

This part of the human entity can only evolve and progress by its own conscious and personal voluntary efforts.

In this, man differs from the animal creation. The animal is able to take care of itself shortly after birth. It inherits, already fully developed, those brain centers for the control of the bodily functions while the newly born human baby must develop slowly and laboriously through patient and persistent effort through the course of many years.

Of voluntary capacities and powers the new-born infant possesses little more than the simplest unicellular animalcule, that is, about all it can do is to scent and swallow food. Its cerebral hemispheres are as yet blank slates, to be inscribed gradually by its conscious and voluntary exertions. Before it can think, reason, speak, walk, or do anything, it must first develop in its brain special centers for every one of those voluntary faculties and functions.

Through these persistent and personal efforts, reason, will, and self-control are gradually evolved and developed; while the animal, being already hereditarily endowed with the faculties and functions necessary for the maintenance of life, has no occasion for the development of the higher faculties and powers, and hence it remains an irresponsible automaton, which cannot be held accountable for its actions.

"The mind of the animal is as pertaining to the conditions that would bring the continuation of species and of foods, and in that manner all in the animal kingdom; pertaining then, Mind and Spirit, men reaching that development wherein the soul becomes the individual that may become the companion, and One with the Creator." 900-31

For:

"...as seen, each animal, each bird, each fowl,

has been so named for some peculiarity of that
individual beast, bird or fowl, and in this
manner represents some particular phase of
man's development in the earth's plane...
"Not that man develops from the animal, or the
animal develops from the man, but, as has been
given, all beasts, all birds, all fowls were
made for man's use and sustenance. Hence, each
must supply...in its associations and relations, some element that is necessary for men's
development." 294-87

"As given, again all manner of animal on the
earth, in the air, under the sea, has been
tamed of man, yet man himself has not reached
that wherein he may perfectly control himself,
save making the will One with the Creator, as
man makes the will of the animal one with his.
The control then in trained animals being the
projection in man. The trained mind of those
in natural state, the element as given, Spirit
and Mind, the specie keep life." 900-31

Therefore:

"...the animal man is a creature of habit. But
learn rather from such the lesson, and not
become so much a part of same. For in nature
and in the animal instincts we find only the
expressions of a universal consciousness of
hope, and never of fear--save created by man
in his indulging in the gratification of
material appetites." 2067-1

To recapitulate: Freedom of choice and action
distinguish the human from the animal. In the animal
kingdom, reasoning power and freedom of action move
in the narrow limits of hereditary and instinct, while
man, through his own personal efforts, is capable of
unlimited development, physically, mentally, morally
and spiritually, both here and in the spiritual plane.
We say "physically" advisedly, for in the spiritual

realms, in the life after death, the physical (spiritual-material body is also capable of deteriorating,
or of a much greater refinement and beauty.

Through the right use of his voluntary faculties,
capacities, and powers, man enables himself to become
master of himself and of his destiny.

This two-fold nature of the human entity justifies
the two-fold attitude of body, mind and soul indepen-
dence on the one hand, and the prayerful and faithful
dependence upon that mysterious intelligent power which
flows into us from the unconscious and controls us
through the sympathetic nervous system. On the other
hand, the conscious mind has voluntary dominion of the
cerebro-spinal system and its various faculties and
capacities as well as the power which nature endowed
us with.

It is our privilege and our duty to maintain both
attitudes, the dependent as well as the independent,
the personal as the impersonal, as well as the desire
and will to plan and to choose, as to perform and to
create. But for the power to execute we are independent, yet dependent upon a higher source. Such may
also be said of man's dependence on one another, yet
each entity is entirely independent of each other.

> "Others are not only dependent upon you, you
> are dependent upon others--in every phase of
> thy experience. For ye are a part of the whole
> experience, and ye add to or detract, according
> to thy own attitude." 1467-16

> "Each individual is an entity, a world in
> itself, yet each entity is dependent one upon
> another. Yet each in their own way expressing
> in their lives that which has become the all-
> possessing idea or ideal to that individual...."
> 290-1

However:

> "Then in preparing self as a portion of a
> group, not independent--but not dependent upon
> any member of the group--be dependent upon God.

In the dependence as is put in individual's falls short." 262-2

Therefore:

"Seek the Lord while He may be found, and then apply just plain everyday judgement to the disturbances of this body. Ye will find that ye will grow in grace, in knowledge, in understanding. And this means in all phases of thy life. For what is the first promise? Know that the Lord thy God is One Lord. That means of soul, of mind and of body. That when the soul, the image of the Creator, is attuned to the divine, you are on the road to meeting thy own self and all will be well with thee." 3174-1

CHAPTER FIFTEEN

THE LAWS OF CURE

This brings us to the consideration of acute inflammatory and feverish diseases. From what has been said, it follows that inflammation and fever are not primary, but secondary manifestations of disease. There cannot arise any form of inflammatory disease in the system unless there is present some enemy to health which nature is endeavoring to overcome and get rid of. On this fact in nature is based the fundamental law of cure.

"Give me fever and I can cure every disease." Thus Hippocrates, the "Father of Medicine," expressed the fundamental law of cure over two thousand years ago. We can express this same law in the following sentence: "Every acute disease is the result of an attempt of the cleansing and healing effort of nature."

This law, when thoroughly understood and applied to the treatment of diseases, will in time do for medical science what the discovery of other natural laws has done for physics, astronomy, chemistry and other exact sciences. It will transform the medical empiricism and confusion of the past and present into an exact science by demonstrating the unity of disease and treatment.

Applying the laws in a general way, it means that all acute diseases, from a simple cold to measles, scarlet fever, diphteria, smallpox, pneumonia, etc., represent nature's efforts to repair injury or to remove from the system some kind of morbid matter, virus and poison, or any other micro-organism dangerous to health and life. From the Cayce readings:

"Toxins that should be eliminated through their proper channels are surcharging tissue and bringing distress to various parts of the body --joints, muscular forces; especially in head

and neck and in ligaments to locomotion at times...

"As the cycle of vibration changes in the cellular body for use of certain portions, the attack comes to the weaker part...

"The centers involved directly are the 10th and 11th dorsal. These feed the tissue and nerve to the intestinal tract, so that the system has gradually come to absorb these toxins from same...they are being carried in the circulation and distributed to various parts of the body.

"The intestinal condition, near the Peyer's glands, is the origin. This in turn has effected the pneumogastric and hypogastric centers, until the hepatic circulation through kidneys has become involved.

"Hence the glands in tonsils and thyroids have become involved producing local conditions."
4517-1

"The disturbance in the eliminations, the tendency for the lack of removing the poisons and toxic forces from the body is bringing about the effects of pressures in the nerves of the locomotories." 1612-4

"Begin with the activities in the diet that will make for the resuscitating of more vital forces. Do not overfeed, so that the body becomes a dross pit--as it were; but only take sufficient that the body does assimilate, does use up those forces that are taken into the system." 626-1

"As we find. there are considerable improvement in the general condition of the body. The lack of fever or temperature indicates the assimilation of those precautionary measures (or substance) that have been taken, and their activity with the general reactions in the system. The lack of discolorations in portions of the arm indicates an improvement also."
670-2

In other words, acute diseases cannot develop in a perfectly normal and healthy body living under conditions favorable to human life. The question may be asked: "If acute diseases represent nature's healing efforts, why is it that people die from them." The answer to this is: the vitality may be too low, the injury or morbid encumbrance too great, or the treatment may be inadequate or harmful, so that nature loses the fight; still, the acute disease represents an effort of nature to overcome the enemies of health and life and to re-establish normal and healthy conditions.

It is a most curious fact that this fundamental principle of natural healing and law of nature has been acknowledged and verified by medical science. The most advanced works on pathology admit the constructive and beneficial character of inflammation. However, when it comes to the treatment of acute diseases, many physicians seem to forget entirely this basic principle of pathology, and treat inflammation and fever as though they were in themselves, inimical and destruc tive to health and life.

From this inconsistency in theory and practice arise all the errors of allopathic medical treatment. Failure to understand this fundamental law of cure accounts for all the confusion on the part of the exponents of the different schools of healing sciences, and for the greater part of human suffering.

The natural healing philosophy never loses sight of the fundamental law of cure. While allopathy regards acute disease conditions as in themselves harmful and hostile to health and life; as something to be "cured" (suppressed should be the word) by drug or knife. The natural healing school of cure regards these forcible cleanings as beneficial and necessary, so long, at least, as people will continue to disregard nature's laws. While, through its simple, natural methods of treatment, natural healing easily modifies the course of inflammatory and feverish processes and keeps them wihtin safe limits. It never checks or suppresses these acute reactions by poisonous drugs, serums, antiseptics, surgical operations, suggestion, or any other suppressive treatment.

Skin eruptions, boils, ulcers, catarrhs, diarrheas, and all other forms of inflammatory febrile
disease conditions are indications that there is something hostile to life and health in the body by which
nature is trying to remove or overcome by these so-
called acute diseases. What, then, can be gained by
suppressing them with poisonous drugs and surgical
operations? Such practice does not allow nature to
carry on her work of cleansing and repair to attain her
ends. The morbid matter which she endeavored to remove
by acute reactions is thrown back into the system.
Worse than that, drug poisons are added to the disease
poisons. Is it any wonder that fatal complications
arise, or that the acute condition is changed to a
chronic disease?

No matter how learned a man may be, if he begins
a problem in arithmetic with the proposition 2X2=5, he
never will arrive at a correct solution if he continues
to figure well into eternity. Neither can allopathy
solve the problem of disease and cure so long as its
basic concept of disease is based on error.

The fundamental law of cure explains why that
the great majority of allopathic prescriptions contain
virulent poisons in some form or another, and why
surgical operations are in high favor with those disciples of modern medicine.

The answer of allopathy to the question, "Why do
you give poisons?" usually is, "Our materia medica
contains poisons because drug poison kills and eliminates disease poisons." However, the claim that drug
poisons merely serve to paralyze vital forces, whereby
the deceptive results of allopathic treatments are
obtained.

The following will explain this more fully. We
have learned that so-called acute diseases are nature's
cleansing and healing efforts. All acute reactions
represent increased activity of vital force, resulting
in feverish and inflammatory conditions, accompanied
by pain, redness, swelling, high temperature, rapid
pulse, catarrhal discharges, skin eruptions, boils
and ulcers.

Allopathy regards these violent activities of

vital force as detrimental and harmful in themselves.
Anything which will inhibit the action of vital force
will, in allopathic parlance, cure (?) acute diseases.
As a matter of fact, nothing more effectively paralyzes
vital force and impairs the vital organs than poisonous
drugs. These, therefore, must necessarily constitute
the favorite means of cure (?) of the regular school
of medicine.

This school mistakes effect for cause. It fails
to see that the local inflammation arising within the
organism is not the disease, but merely denotes the
locality and the method through which nature is trying
her best to discharge the morbid encumbrances; that
the acute reaction is local, but that its causes or
feeders are always constitutional and must be treated
constitutionally. When, under the influence of the
rational, natural treatment, the poisonous irritants
are eliminated from the blood and tissues, the local
symptoms take care of themselves; it does not matter
whether they manifest as pimple or cancer, as a simple
cold or pneumonia, or as in the following reading for
person # 3886-1 given March 2, 1930. The prognosis--
anemia:

> *"Mr. C: Yes, we have the body here, (3886).*
> *Now, we find there are disorders of specific*
> *natures as cause the disturbance with the phy-*
> *sical forces of the body. These have to do*
> *with the assimilations in the system. Hence*
> *that tenseness as is seen in the system through*
> *the building or replenishing forces, and ten-*
> *dency towards anemic forces in the general*
> *system.*
> *IN THE BLOOD SUPPLY--*
> *"This somewhat below normal in the re-building,*
> *and kept so by those conditions of a specific*
> *nature as exist in the region of the lacteal*
> *ducts. There the inflammation is produced.*
> *From that source comes that distress as is*
> *seen in liver, and the temperature as is*
> *produced in the upper portion of system, and*
> *the sudden changes as come, and the nausea as*

comes. These produced from that inflammation
as has existed from congestion, or from cold,
that has produced in the intestinal tract that
inflammation of the mucous membrane of the
digestive system, centering most about this
portion. Then the indigestion, the activities
in the colon, through the activity of the emunctory and lymphatic circulation, becoming
involved. This raising the exterior circulation.

"IN THE NERVE FORCES--these very good, save
when such inflammation produces that condition
in the centers of the sympathetic, as   to
cause that irrational forces as come from nerve
forces--that is, in the nerve themselves--not
the mental forces of the body.

"IN THE FUNCTIONING ORGANS--these, as seen,
function under the stress of those conditions
as produced there. There will also be found
that a lesion--of a minor nature, apparently
exists in the 8th and 9th dorsal. This produced
as much by the system attempting to adjust
itself. through the supplying of energy to the
system from this portion, as from the first
cause--where there was the wrench, or the
depression there.

"In meeting, then, the needs of these--for
unless these are corrected, we may find disorders may occur, especially through any of
the system where the ducts, or the non-activity
--as in the portion of the kidney, or in the
portion of the system about the appendix
region, or in the cavity itself in lower
portion of the intestine, and also that in
throat, bronchia, and upward. These are inflammation centers from which the conditions may
spread, unless elimnated from the system. The
body is very good at times, at others the
temperature rising, and the distress in the
assimilation produces this distraughtness
throughout.

"In meeting the needs, then, at the present--

first consideration should be given to that
as regarding that which may be assimilated by
the system, and still not produce irritation
to any of the mucous membranes, either in the
stomach or in the duodenum, or in any portion
of the intestinal tract. These, we would find,
will not be used--not too much of milk, unless
it was goat's milk. These would be very good,
goat's milk especially.

"In the applications for the conditions themselves, we should keep the body quiet. Keep
an antiseptic in the system that is alkaline
in its reaction. We would correct these conditions in the dorsal region, and we would
keep those of the system as coordinating
through the activity of the nerve energy, and
through that portion of the system where the
activities come with those of the locomotaries,
especially. We may use small quantities of
spirits fermenti, if the alcohol is burned
from same. This will ease, and even reduce
temperature in the body.

"Massage each day, along the whole of the
cerebro-spinal system. with those of Olive Oil
Myrrh, and Sassafras Oil--equal parts. Following same when temperature arises, with those
of the alcohol, as will reduce the temperature.
This applied externally. Those of the antiseptic internally, we would use those of the
Glyco. We would also use those of an oil enema
to reduce temperature in intestinal system,
and to assist in carrying the refuse from the
system without producing too much irritation.
Do that.

"The food values, as we should see, should be
those of citrus fruit juices, or vegetable
juices, and occasionally--taken more as medicine than as food--those of beef juice. We will
build the system back to a normal condition.
This should not require more than ten days to
two weeks, to be near normal.

"Do this, and we will find we will bring the

normal conditions for this body.
"In making the adjustments as will be neces-
sary, and in reducing the temperature as will
be necessary with the manipulation and massage
--these should not be done too severe, but
just quiet--and to stimulate the system, and
so as to relieve those distresses as come from
the inflammation in the region here, or in the
ducts--as has been given.
"We are through for the present." 3886-1

Everywhere in nature there rules the great law
of action and reaction. All life sways back and forth
between giving and receiving, and between action and
reaction. The very breath of life mysteriously comes
and goes in rhytmical flow. So also heaves and falls
in ebb and tide the bosom of Mother Earth.

In some of its aspects, this law is called the
Law of Dual Effect. On its action depends the preservation of energy.

The Great Master expressed the ethical application of this law when He said: "Give, and it shall be
given unto you...."

In the realms of physical nature, giving and
receiving, action and reaction balance each other
mechanically and automatically. What we gain in power
we lose in speed or volume, and vice-a-versa. It then
makes it possible for the mechanics, the scientists.
and the astronomers to predict with great mathematical
precision for ages in advance the results of certain
activities in nature.

The great law of dual effect forms the foundation
of the healing sciences. It is related to and governs
every phenomena of health, disease and cure. When
formulated, the fundamental law of cure can be stated
in the words: "Every acute disease is the result of a
healing effort of nature," and this is but another
expression of the great law of action and reaction.
What we commonly call crisis, acute reaction, or acute
disease, is in reality nature's attempt to establish
a healthy body.

Applied to the physical activity of the body,

the law of compensation may be expressed as follows: "Every agent affecting the human organism produces two effects--a first, apparent, temporary effect, and a second, lasting effect. The secondary, lasting effect is always contrary to the primary, transient effect."

For instance: the first and temporary effect of cold water applied to the skin consists in sending the blood to the interior; but in order to compensate for the local depletion, nature responds by sending greater quantities of blood back to the surface, resulting in increased warmth and better surface circulation.

The first effect of a hot bath is to draw blood to the surface; but the secondary effect sends the blood back to the interior, leaving the surface bloodless and chilled.

Stimulants, therefore, produce their deceptive effects by burning up the reserve stores of vital energy in the organism. This is inevitably followed by weakness and exhaustion in exact proportion to the previous excitation.

The primart effect of relaxation and sleep is weakness, numbness, and death-like stupor; while the secondary effect, however, is an increase of vitality.

The law of dual effect governs all drug action. The first, temporary, violent effect of poisonous drugs, when given in physiological doses, is usually due to nature's efforts to overcome and eliminate these substances. The secondary, lasting effect is due to the retention of the drug poisons in the system and their action on the organism itself.

In theory and practice, allopathy considers the first effect only, and ignores the after-effects of drugs and surgical operations. It administers remedies whose first effect is contrary to the disease condition. Therefore, in accordance with the law of action and reaction, the secondary and lasting effects of such remedies must be similar or like the disease condition existent in the human body.

Common, every day experience should teach us that this is so, for laxatives and cathartics always tend to produce chronic conditions of constipation.

The secondary effect of stimulants and tonics of

any kind is increased weakness, and their continued use often results in complete exhaustion and paralysis of mental and physical powers.

Headache pills, pain killers, opiates, sedatives and hypnotics may paralyze the brain and nerves into temporary insensibility; but, if due to constitutional causes, the pain, nervousness and insomnia will always return with redoubled force. If taken habitually all of these agents invariably tend to create heart disease and paralysis, and ultimately develop into the "dope addict."

Cold and catarrh cures, as are now available on the market, suppress nature's efforts to eliminate waste and morbid matter through the mucous linings of the respiratory tract, and drive the disease matter back into the lungs, this breeding pneumonia, chronic catarrhs, asthma and influenza.

Mercury, Iodine and all other alteratives, by suppression of external elimination, create internal chronic diseases of the most dreadful types.

So the recital might be continued all through orthodox materia medica. Each drug breeds its own peculiar new disease symptoms which are in turn cured (?) by other poisons, until the insane asylum or merciful death rings down the curtain on a tragic ruined life.

The teaching and the practice of Homeopathy, as explained in another chapter, is fully in harmony with the law of action and reaction. Acting upon the basic principle of homeopathy: that "like cures like," and administers remedies whose first, temporary effect is similar to the disease condition. In accordance with the law of dual effect, then, the secondary effect of these remedies must be contrary to the condition of disease, that is, curative.

The law of cure is dependent, of course, on the knowledge that we cannot serve two masters, for there is ever before us the matter of choice.

> "...as given by the Father--there cannot be the full consciousness of the one without the laying aside of the other, for no one serves two master." 900-328

"Walk, then, in the light that is set by self as the ideal. Ye cannot serve God and mannom. Ye will be enjoined one to the other. Keep thine counsel in many things. Be a good listener, and an excellent worker." 311-8

Therefore:

"There is set before thee two ways, ever, and the choice is given to a soul as to whether it chooses that in keeping with the ideals set in Creative influences, or God, making the will one with, not blaming Him with that which comes to self, but self--as to what has been builded and what self does about His love, law, and experience--in every relation." 347-2

CHAPTER SIXTEEN

NATURAL DIETETICS

The chemical composition of blood and lymph depends upon the chemical compositions of food and drink, and upon the normal or the abnormal condition of the digestive system.

The purer the food and drink, the less it contains of morbid matter and the poison-producing materials, and the more it contains of the elements necessary for the proper execution of the manifold functions of the organism. In the building and repair of tissues, and the neutralization and elimination of waste and systematic poisons, the more "natural," the more "normal" the function of the diet will be.

The system of dietetics as given in the Edgar Cayce readings is based mostly on the consumption of raw and fresh vegetables, which are the only perfect natural food combinations that should be eaten raw, and preferably as salads.

In their composition, vegetables build correspondingly healthy, red, arterial blood and contains all of the elements which the new-born and growing organism needs in the right combinations, providing, of course, that the vegetables were raised in good health, or without the benefit of chemical fertilizers, or sprays of insecticides. But more importantly, that is, grown in the area where the body resides.

Much of the information in this chapter is drawn mostly from Cayce's enormous stock of information on this subject, and if more material is needed, it is suggested that you avail yourself of the opportunity to research this information that was given from the psychic realm through the channel Edgar Cayce.

Normal diet:

"Normal diet...use at least three vegetables

*that grow above the ground to one that grows
under the ground."* 3371-1

*"Be mindful that there is at least one meal
each day taken of raw green vegetables; this
doesn't mean green in color only but those
that are raw and fresh, not stale vegetables.*
906-1

*"There is no supplementary to green foods in
the real way or manner; though if there are
the periods when there is not the ability to
obtain or have the green foods...these others
may be used, but rather as extremities than
as a regular activity in same, see?"* 1158-11

*"These (referring to vegetable supplements)
may be taken if there is a lack of those
activities from the raw salad; but they do
not, WILL not, supply the energies as well or
as efficaciously for the BODY as if there were
the efforts made to have at least one meal
each day altogether of raw vegetables, or two
meals carrying a raw salad as a portion of
same—each day."* 1158-18

However:

*"All such properties (as vitamins) that add
to the system are more efficacious if they are
given for periods, left off for periods and
begun again. For if the system comes to rely
upon such influences wholly it ceases to produce the vitamins even though the food values
may be kept normally balanced.*
*"And it's much better that these be produced
in the body from the normal development than
supplied mechanically, for nature is much better yet than science!*
*"This we find then, given twice a day for two
or three weeks, left off for a week and then
begun again, especially through the winter
months, would be much more effective with
the body."* 759-12

Therefore, if any food combination or diet is to be "normal" or "natural," it must approach in its chemical composition the nutrients needed to produce healthy, red arterial blood. This does furnish a very strict scientific basis for an exact science of dietetics, and proves true not only in the chemical aspect of the diet problem, but also in its balance and its relationship to most every other aspect of practical application.

The regular school of medicine pays little or no attention to rational food regulation or balance. In fact it knows mostly nothing about it, because natural dietetics are not yet taught, even today, in any of the medical schools.

As a result of this condition, the dietary advice given by old school practioners is something like as follows: "Eat what agrees with you; plenty of good, nourishing food. There is nothing in diet fads. What is one man's meat is another man's poison, etc., etc.

However, if we study nutrition from a scientific point of view, we cannot but help find that certain foods, and among these, especially the highly-valued flesh foods, eggs, sugar and white flour, create in the system large quantities of morbid and poisonous substances, while on the other hand, vegetables and fruits, which are rich in the organic salts, tend to neutralize and eliminate from the system all of the waste material and poisons created in the processes of protein and starch digestion.

The accumulation of waste and systemic poison is the cause of the majority of diseases arising within the human organism. Therefore it is imperative that the neutralizing and eliminating food elements found in raw vegetables be provided in sufficient quantities.

"Beware in the diet of sugars, starches of those that produce same." 119-1

"The tendencies for too much starches, pastries, white bread should be almost eliminated ...They are not very good for the body in any form." 416-18

> *"Do not combine too much starches, nor too much of any of those things that will create too great a quantity of alcoholic reaction-- such as candies withANY of the starches; these produce that reaction with the system of the CHARACTER of fermentation that produces an alcoholic reaction disturbing to the system."*
> *1315-7*

Also:

> *"Beware of excessive acid-producing foods; though it must be considered that the body in its developing stage requires sufficient of those energies from sugars that are proper for the system. Hence the sweets should be of such natures that they do not form a character of acid that becomes detrimental to those very tendencies that are being overcome..." 795-4*

On this fact turns the entire problem of natural dietetics. For the old school of medicine looks upon starches and sweets, fats and proteins as the only elements of nutrition worthy of consideration.

In this volume we cannot go into the full details of the dietary question. This will be found in some volumes now on the market dealing with the question of "Natural Diets." However, we state here in a general way that in the treatment of chronic diseases, with very few exceptions, that a strict vegetarian diet is favored for the reason that most all chronic diseases are created, as previously stated, by that accumulation of the "feces of the cells" in the body.

Every morsel of animal flesh is saturated with these excrements of the cells in the form of uric acid as well as many other kinds of acids, "alkaloids of putrefaction," ptomaines, etc. The organism of the meat-eater must dispose not only of its own impurities produced in the processes of digestion and of cell-metabolism, but also of the morbid substances as are already contained within the animal's dead flesh.

Since the cure of chronic diseases consists so largely in purifying the body of morbid materials, it stands to reason that a "chronic" must cease taking these in his daily food. To do otherwise would be like sweeping the dirt out of the house through the front door and carrying it in again through the back door.

Whether one approves of strict vegetarism as a continuous mode of living or not, it will be admitted that the change from a meat diet to a non-meat diet must be of great benefit in the treatment of chronic diseases. The readings recommend the following:

"In the diet keep away from red meats, ham, or rare steak or roast. Rather use fish, fowl and lamb..." 3596-1

"Avoid too much of the heavy meats not well cooked. Eat plenty of vegetables of all characters. The meats taken would be preferably fish, fowl and lamb; others not so often. Breakfast bacon, crisp, may be taken occasionally." 1710-4

However:

"Meats of certain characters are necessary in the body-building forces in this system, and should not be wholly abstained from in the present. Spiritualize those influences, those activities, rather than abstaining. For, as He gave, that which cometh out--rather than that which goeth in--defileth the spiritual body." 295-10

"This, to be sure, is not an attempt to tell the body to go back to eating meat, but do supply, then, through the body forces, supplements, either in vitamins or in substitutes, for those who would hold to these influences --but purifying of mind is of the mind, not of the body. For, as the Master gave, it is not that which entereth in the body, but that which cometh out that causes sin. It is what one does with the purpose, for all things are

pure in themselves, and are for the sustenance
of man, body, mind, and soul, and remember--
these must work together..." 5401-1

The cure of chronic conditions depend upon the radical changes in the cells and tissues of the body, as explained in a former chapter. The old, abnormal, faulty diet will continue to build the same abnormal and disease-encumbered tissues. The more thorough and radical the change in diet toward normalcy and purity, the quicker the cells and tissues of the body will change toward the more normal and thus bring about a complete regeneration of the organism.

Anything short of this may be palliative treatment but it is not worthy of the name "cure."

This phase of the diet question will now follow in the next few pages.

The outline of a "natural diet" regimen, which has been found by experience to meet all requirements of an healthy organism, even when people have to work very hard physically or mentally, follows.

However, in case of disease, certain modifications may have to be made according to individual needs. Persons in a low, negative state, whether physical, mental, or emotional, may temporarily require the addition of certain flesh foods to their diet.

In the accompanying table we have divided all food materials into five main groups:

Group 1----starches (carbohydrates)

Group 2----dextrines and sugars (carbohydrates)

Group 3----fats and oils (hydrocarbons)

Group 4----white of egg, lean meat, gluten of grains and pulses, proteins of nuts, milk. (protein)

Group 5----iron, sodium, calcium, potassium, magnesium, silicon. These are contained in large amounts in juicy fruits and leafy, juicy vegetables (organic minerals).

As a general rule, let one-half of your food consists of Group 5, and the other half of a mixture of the first four groups.

If you wish to follow an absolute pure-food diet, exclude meat, fish, fowl, meat soups and sauces, and

all other foods prepared from the dead flesh of animals.
    This is brief and comprehensive (which is really our intention). So let us begin.

Smoking and drinking:

Do not use coffee, tea, alcoholic or carbonated beverages, tobacco, or stimulants of any kind.

"Q.- Have personal vices as tobacco and whiskey any influence on one's health or longevity?
"A.- As just has been indicated, you are suffering from the use of some of these in the present; but it is over-indulgence. In moderation these are not too bad, but man so seldom will be moderate. Or, as most say, those who even indulge will make themselves pigs, but we naturally are pigs when there is over-indulgence. This, of course, makes for conditions which are to be met. For what one sows that must one reap. This is unchangeable law."
                                        5233-1
"Q.- Is the moderate use of liquor, tobacco and meat a bar to spiritual growth?
"A.- For this entity, yes. For some, no."
                                        2981-1
"Q.- Does smoking hurt the body?
"A.- Moderation, not so harmful as would be the nerve and mental reaction from total abstinence from same." 1568-2

"Q.- Would smoking be detrimental to me or beneficial?
"A.- This depends very much upon self. In moderation, smoking is not harmful; but to a body that holds such as being out of line with its best mental or spiritual unfoldment, do not smoke." 2981-2

However:

"No beer, no strong drink; though red wine as

a food may be taken occasionally--for this is blood building and blood-resisting forces are carried in same--as iron and those plasms that make for the proper activity upon the system. But never more than two or two and a half ounces of same, but this only with black or brown bread, and not with sweets." 1308-1

"...wine taken in excess--of course--is harmful; wine taken with bread alone is body, blood and nerve and brain building." 821-1

"A stimulation occasionally as of wine with bread, not as a drink but just as a potion to bring rest to the body. When taken it should only be with rye or sour or brown bread."
846-1
"Give beef juices and liquids, foods that are very stimulating. Every form of better stimulant that is for building strength, as wine. These especially, with the fish foods."
2074-2

Coffee and tea:

"Q.- Will coffee hurt the body?
"A.- Coffee without cream or milk is not so harmful..." 1568-2

"Q.- Is coffee good? If so, how often?
"A.- Coffee taken properly is a food value.
"To many conditions, as with this body, the caffeine in same is hard upon the digestion; especially when there is the tendency for a plethora condition in the lower end of the stomach.
"Hence the use of coffee or the chicory in the food values that arise from the combinations of coffee with breads or meats or sweets is helpful.
"But for this body, it is preferable that the tannin be mostly removed. Then it can be taken two to three times a day, but without milk or cream." 404-6

"Q.- Are tea and coffee harmful?
"A.- For this body tea is preferable to coffee,
but in excess is hard upon the digestion. To
be sure, it should never be taken with milk."
1622-1

"Q.- Is tea and coffee harmful to the body?
"A.- Tea is more harmful than coffee. Any nerve
reaction is more susceptible to the character
of tea that is usually found in this country,
though in some manners in which it is produced
it would be well. Coffee, taken properly, is
a food; that is, without cream or milk."
303-2

However:

"...coffee is as of those properties as stimu-
lants to the nerve system. The dross from
same is caffeine, and is not digestible in
the system, and must necessarily then be
eliminated. When such are allowed to remain
in the colon there is thrown off from same
poisons. Eliminated as it is in this system,
coffee is a food value, and is preferable to
many stimulants that might be taken, see?"
294-86

It is stated, therefore, that moderation is the key in the consumption of tea and coffee, also alcoholic beverages should be avoided, excepting wine and only if taken in moderation.

Instead of the customary coffee, tea, or cocoa, delicious drinks, which are nutritious but yet non-stimulating, may be prepared from the many different fruit and vegetable juices. They may be served cold in hot weather and warm in winter. Recipes for fruit and vegetable juices can be found in any cookbook.

If more suitable drinks are desired, white of an egg may be added, or the entire egg may be used in combination with prune juice, fig juice, or any of the other acid fruit juices. Other desirable and unobjectional additions to beverages are flaked nuts, or a small banana blended to a liquid in the blender.

The juice of a lemon or an orange, unsweetened,

diluted with twice the amount of water taken on rising
is one of the best means of purifying the blood and
other fluids of the body and, incidentally helps to
clear the complexion. The water in which prunes and
figs have been cooked should be taken freely to remedy
any constipation problems.

It is indicated in the Cayce readings that more
of the products grown in the same area where the body
lives should be consumed. This is known as "Acclimi-
tization."

*"Have vegetables that are fresh and especi-
ally those grown in the vicinity where the
body resides.*
"Shipped vegetables are never very good."
                                    2-14
*"Do not have large quantities of any fruits,
vegetables, meats—which are not grown in or
that do not come from the area where the body
is—at the time it partakes of such foods.*
*"This will be found to be a good rule to be
followed by all. This prepares the system to
acclimate itself to any given territory."*
                                    3542-1

Therefore:

*"As indicated, use more of the products of the
soil that are grown in the immediate vicinity.
These are better for the body than any specific
set of fruits, vegetables, grasses or what
not. We should add more of the original sources
of proteins." 4047-1*

*"The diet we would change only as there are the
seasonal conditions, of course; the fruits and
vegetables that are seasonal, and especially
of the district in which the body resides—
these use." 2084-6*

Also:

"The climatic conditions here are not the basis

of the trouble. The body can adjust itself. As we have indicated, bodies can usually adjust themselves to climatic conditions if they adhere to the diet and activities, and all characters of foods that are produced in the area where they reside. This will more quickly adjust a body to any particular area or climate than any other thing." 4047-1

Acid and alkaline balance:

"Q.- What should the diet be?
"A.- Those things that will not create too much of an acid, or too much of an alkaline condition throughout the system. Rather be the alkaline than acid--never allowing the system to become over-taxed by not having the proper condition in intestinal tract. Those that are in keeping with such, see? Common good judgement, according to that which agrees and disagrees with the body, see?" 140-12

"Q.- What foods are acid forming for this body?
"A.- All of those that are combining fats with sugars. Starches naturally are inclined for acid reaction. But a normal diet is about twenty percent acid to eighty percent alkaline producing." 1523-3

"...have rather a percentage of eighty percent alkaline-producing to twenty percent acid-producing foods.
"Then it is well that the body not become as one that couldn't do this, that or the other; or a slave to an idea of a set diet." 1568-2

"As indicated, keep a tendency for alkalinity in the diet. This does not necessitate that there should never be any of the acid-forming foods included in the diet; for an over-alkalinity is much more harmful than a little tendency occasionally for acidity. But remem-

ber there are those tendencies in the system
for cold and congestion to affect the body,
and cold cannot, does not, exist in alkalines."
808-3

"The diet should be more body-building; that
is, less acid foods and more of the alkaline-
reacting will be the better in these directions.
Milk and all its products should be a portion
of the body's diet now; also those food values
carrying an easy assimilation of iron, silicon,
and those elements or chemicals--as all forms
of berries, most of the vegetables of a leafy
nature. Fruits and vegetables, nuts and the
like, should form a greater part of the regular
diet in the present..." 480-19

Therefore:

"...when there is the tendency towards an
alkaline system there is less effect of cold
and congestion." 270-33

Next to the leafy vegetables, fruits and berries
are the most valuable foods of the "organic minerals"
group. Lemons, grapefruits, oranges, apples are most
beneficial as blood purifiers. Plums, pears, peaches,
apricots, cherries, grapes, etc., contain large amounts
of fruit sugars in easily assimilable forms and are
also very valuable on account of their mineral salts.
The different kinds of berries are even richer
in mineral salts than the acid and sub-acid fruits.
In the old country homes they are always at hand either
dried or preserved to serve during the winter months,
not only as delicious food supplements, but also as
valuable home remedies.
Fruits and berries are best eaten raw, although
they may be stewed or baked. Very few people know that
rhubard and cranberries are very palatable when cut
up fine and well mixed with honey, being allowed to
stand for about an hour before serving. Prepared in
this way, they require much less sweetening and therefore do not tax the organism nearly as much as the

ordinary rhubarb or cranberry sauce, which usually contains an excessive amount of sugar.

It is better to cook apples, cranberries, rhubarb, strawberries, and all other acid fruits without sugar until soft, and to add the sugar afterwards. Much less sugar will be required to sweeten sufficiently than when the sugar is added before or during the cooking. As for apples, Cayce had this to say:

"We would use first the apple diet to purify the system; that is, for three days eat nothing but apples of the Jonathan variety....The Jonathan is usually grown farther north than the Delicious, but these are of the same variety, but eat some. You may drink coffee if you desire, but do not put milk or cream in it, especially while you are taking the apples. "At the end of the third day, the next morning take about two tablespoonsful of Olive Oil."
                                    780-12

"No raw apples; or if raw apples are taken, take them and nothing else--three days of raw apples only, and then Olive Oil, and we will cleanse all toxic forces from any system."
                                    820-2

Dried fruits ranks next to the fresh in value, as the evaporating process only removes a large percentage of water, without changing the chemical composition of the fruits in any way. Prunes, apricots, apples, pears, peaches, and berries may be obtained in the dried state all through the year. Dates, figs, raisins, and currants also come under this heading.

Cayce recommends a combination of dried dates, figs and corn meal as being uplifting spiritually.

"And for this especial body (a mixture of) dates, figs, (that are dried) cooked with a little corn meal (a very little sprinkled in) then this taken with milk, should be almost a spiritual food for the body..." 275-45

"Q.- Any further suggestions for maintaining maximum health...?

"A.- Do these, as we find the better conditions for the body.
"It is well for this body, or growing bodies,
or elderly individuals also, for strength
building and for correcting the eliminations,
to use this as a cereal, or a small quantity
of this with the cereal, or it may be served
with milk or cream.
"Secure the unpitted Syrian or Black Figs and
the Syrian Dates. Cut or grind very fine, a
cup of each. Put them in a double boiler with
just a little goat's milk in same--a tablespoonful of Yellow Corn Meal." 1188-10

"...equal portions of black figs or Assyrian
Figs and Assyrian Dates--these ground together
or cut very fine, and to a pint of such a
combination put half a handful of corn meal or
crushed wheat. These cooked together."274-45

Therefore:

"As the soul seeks, then, for that which is
the sustenance of the body, as what the food
is to a developing, a growing body, so are
the words of truth (which are life, which are
love, which are God) sought that make for
growth, even as the digesting of the material
things in a body makes for a growth. This
growth may not be felt in the consciousness
of materialization. It is experienced by the
consciousness of the soul, by which it enables
the soul to use the attributes of the soul's
food, even as the growth of the body makes for
the use of the muscular forces or attributes
of the physical body." 254-68

"For the body finds that while spiritual
thought and spiritual food values are essen-
tially supplying elements to a physical body,
in the material plane it is necessary also that
material food values be taken for sustaining

*not only the physical forces but the spiritual
elements as well; to keep them in contact or
as parallel one to another in their activity.
"So it is with all force and influence or
activity in a physical body." 516-4*

*"Foods of the spirit are as necessary to the
mental well-being as the carnal forces of foods
for the maintaining of an equilibrium in the
physical body." 274-3*

*"The body mental and spiritual needs spiritual
food-prayer, meditation, thinking upon spiritual things. For the body is indeed the temple
of the living God. Treat it as such, physically and mentally." 4008-1*

Milk:

It is suggested that milk should be a part of the
natural diet, because milk in its chemical composition,
is the only perfect natural food combination extent.
Naturally, the question arises: "Why, then, not live
on milk entirely?" To this is replied: While milk is
the natural food for the new-born and growing infant,
it is not natural for the adult as such. The digestive
apparatus of the infant is especially adapted to the
digestion of milk, while that of the adult requires
more of the solid and bulky foods.
Milk is very beneficial as an article of diet in
all acid diseases, because it contains comparatively
low percentages of carbohydrates and proteins and yet
have large amounts of organic salts.

*"For milk, whether it is the dry or the pas-
teurized or raw, is near to the perfect combination of forces for the human comsumption."*
1703-2
*"...milk in all its forms, and the products of
same should be a portion of the diet..."*
480-42
"...well that the general strength be builded

up with beef juices, eggs and milk drinks, and the easily assimilated foods." 265-9

Milk may be taken directly with any sweetish, alkaline fruits, or the dried fruits, such as prunes, dates, raisins, etc. and also, of course, with vegetable salads. With the latter, if taken together with milk, no lemon juice or such should be taken.

All acid and sub-acid fruits should be taken as far away from the meal where milk is a part.

"Orange juice and milk are helpful, but these would be taken at opposite ends of the day; not together." 274-9

"Mornings--Orange juice. Do not take it when cereals are taken that milk is eaten with, though they may be alternated." 418-2

For those whom straight milk does not agree, buttermilk is an excellent food. In many instances a straight buttermilk diet for a certain period of time will prove very beneficial.

"Q.- Is buttermilk good?
"A.- This depends upon the manner in which it is made. This would tend to produce gas if it is the ordinary kind. But that made by the use of the Bulgarian tablets is good, in moderation; not too much." 404-6

"The diet should be that as will best assimilate in and for the system, which of necessity then should be changed often. As much buttermilk as the body will assimilate will always be good for the system." 67-1

"Since the temperature has been allayed, there is the necessity, to be sure, that there are not foods used nor activities that would tend to make for the weakening of the digestive forces, nor the allowing of activities of the

*assimilating system--the liver, the kidneys
or the whole hepatic circulation--to become
so congested as to allow the temperature to
arise again.*
*"Hence we would keep rather a tendency to the
alkaline-producing foods...*
*"To be sure, buttermilk (if it is homemade)
--may be gradually added; not all at once, but
just sufficient that the body gains strength
physically. And keep the eliminations well."*
                                        1409-4

Yogurt:

*"Also we would add yogurt in the diet as an
active cleanser through the colon and intestinal system. This would be most beneficial,
not only purifying the alimentary canal, but
adding the vital forces necessary to enable
those portions of the system to function in
the nearer normal manner.*
*"Thus we may bring the abilities for strength
and for purifying the circulatory forces, upon
which depends the strength to resist physically
the inroads of the infectious forces that
disturb the locomotion as well as the pul-
monary and the circulatory system and the
strength through the depleting of the nerve
energies of the body." 1542-1*

*"Yogurt is prepared by making a curd that
passes through the system to absorb and aid
in the eliminations. Use in milk, then, as a
curd--and take very small sips for the body.*
*"Yogurt is a preparation from honeycomb, you
see, that acts to take casseins from milk that
are injurious to the system and helpful in the
intestinal tract." 1045-8*

*"Evenings--For the most part leafy vegetables,
and not too much of same. Use yogurt in the
evening meal...*
"This is to act as a cleanser for the alimen-

tary canal, as well as a better balance for the fermenting and the eliminations of poisons from the system." 1762-1

"The yogurt in its preparation may make for the greater absorbing influences through the intestinal system, and with the general inactivity keep the coordinations of activities between the circulatory forces of the liver, the spleen, the pancreas, the lungs, the kidneys, more in order. For from such disturb the breaking down of the katabolism becomes the destructive force in any condition of this nature." 1045-9

Honey and milk:

"Honey and milk should be taken as a nightcap, as it were. Stir or dissolve a full teaspoonful of strained honey into a glass or tumbler of heated milk. Taking this about twenty to thirty minutes before retiring will be found to be most helpful, most beneficial." 1539-1

"Also when the osteopathic treatments are begun, but not until then (for the system should be cleansed thoroughly first, by the taking of the two rounds of the properties indicated), we would begin taking each evening before retiring about a cupful of heated milk (raw milk, preferably), in which there would be stirred a level teaspoonful of pure honey. Do not boil the milk, but just let it come to the heating point, and then stir in the honey."
                                                          2057-1

"Eliminating the poisons and the tensions or 'buzz' as it were upon the nerve system, as indicated, will naturally make for easier sleep.
"In the beginning of these, if there is the tendency for sleeplessness, or insomnia, stir a teaspoonful of pure honey in a glass of hot milk and drink same." 2050-1

Sweets:

Honey is a very valuable food and a natural laxative. It is not generally known that honey is not a purely vegetable product, but that in passing through the organism of the bee it partakes of its life element, which is readily transmitted to the person consuming it.

Honey is one of the best forms of sugar available. The white sugar is detrimental to health, because it has become inorganic through the refining process. The brown, unrefined granulated sugar, or maple-sugar, or beet sugar should be used instead.

"Q.-What type of sweets may be eaten by the body?
"A.-Honey, especially in the honeycomb; or preserves made with beet rather than cane sugar. Not too great a quantity of any of these, of course, but the forces in sweets to make for the proper activity through the action of the gastric flows are as necessary as body building (elements); for these become body building in making for the proper fermentation (if it may be called so) in the digestive activities. Hence two or three times a week the honey upon the bread or the food values would furnish that necessary in the whole system." 808-3

"Q.- Suggest best sugars for body?
"A.- Beet sugars are the better for all, or the cane sugars that are not clarified."
                                    1131-2

Therefore:

"Keep the body from too much sweets--though (have) sufficient of sweets to form sufficient alcohol for the system; that is, the kind of sweets, rather than sweets. Grape sugars-- hence jellies, or (sweets) of that nature--are well. Chocolates that are plain, not those of any (brand) that carry corn starches should be taken--or not those that carry too much of the

cane sugars. Grape sugar, or beet sugars, or
(sweets) of that nature may be taken." 307-6

Saccharin:

"Saccharin may be used. Brown sugar is not
harmful. The better would be to use beet sugar
for sweetening." 307-6

The use of beet sugar is preferable to cane;
or still more preferable is saccaharin, as
sweetening." 1963-2

"Q.- How much sweets can the body take?
"A.- If these are of saccharin as their base
eat what the body requires. There will be periods when the body's appetite will desire
these, but supply same not from cane sugar."

889-1

Starches and sweets:

"Do not combine any of the starches with any
quantity of sweets. Do not take food values
that cause great quantity of alcoholic reaction.
This does not refer to alcohol, but sweets and
certain starches produce a character of fermentation that is alcoholic that makes for
excess of fatty portions for the body."

"As has been indicated, these are not to be
entirely tabu, but as would be from a normal
mental balance of consideration, take about
eighty percent alkaline-producing foods to
twenty percent acid-producing. Sugars are in
the MAIN, combined with starches, acid-producing. Starches also produce energy, as does
sugar. It is the combinations of these that
become rather the hindrances than the INDIVI-
DUAL properties themselves, see? 877-28

"Do not take large quantities of sweets at
the same period that starches are taken..."

1023-1

Therefore:

"...in all bodies, the less activities there
are in physical exercise or manual activity,
the greater should be the alkaline-reacting
foods taken. Energies or activities may burn
acids, but those who lead the sedentary life
or the non-active life can't go on sweets or
too much starches--but these should be well-
balanced." 798-1

Starches and meats:

"Rather is it the combination of foods that
make for disturbance with most physical
bodies...
"...avoid combinations where corn, potatoes,
rice, spaghetti or the like are taken all at
the same meal...all of these tend to make for
too great a quantity of starch--especially if
any meat is taken at such a meal...for the
activities of the gastric flow of the digestive
system are the requirements of one reaction in
the gastric flow for starch and another for
protein, or for the activities of the carbohydrates as combined with starches of this
nature...Sweets and meats taken at the same
meal are preferable to starches and meats."
                                        416-9
"Be mindful of the diet, that there are not
the combinations of fat meats with starches.
These make for the use of the varied activities
and cause a superacidity." 1197-1

"In the diet be mindful that there is not too
great a combination of starches, as to form
for the circulatory forces and the digestive
area too great an acidity--which not only
produces the conditions that disturb through
the poor elimination and the toxic forces
through the alimentary canal, but produces in
the blood stream itself the inability--with

*the activities of the properties indicated--
for proper coordination. Twenty percent acid
to eighty percent alkaline-reacting should be
the proper balance.*

*"Do not combine ever any red meats with the
starches, as of white bread or white potatoes,
at the same meal. The meats should consists
principally of fowl, fish or lamb. Not any
fried foods at any time." 1288-1*

Meats: Pork:

*"Here, in the condition of this body, we have
a result of the absorption of certain food
values that arise from eating a certain character of foods.*

*"The character of dross it makes in the body-
functioning causes a fungi that produces in
the system a crystallization of the muscles
and nerves in portions of the body.*

*"These results have been apparent in the pelvic
organs, the whole lumbar-sacral area, portions
of the sciatic nerves, the knees and feet--all
of these are giving distress.*

*"These distresses began as acute pain, rheu-
matic or neuritic. They are closer to neuritic-
arthritic reactions. This is pork--the effect
of same.*

*"Q.- What had the body been eating that it
should not?*

"A.- Meats, in the form of hog meat." 294-41

*"To be sure, there must be kept for the body
properties that will continue to act as an
antiseptic for the lungs, throat, bronchials,
and the constant building up of the blood
supply; but no hog meats should ever be taken
by the body--not even hog liver!" 4874-3*

*"Keep away from any meats, especially hog
meats. A little fish or fowl may be taken.*

*"Q.- Will this treatment if carefully carried
out give permanent cure?*

"A.- This will depend upon the body's returning
to those things that would bring back the
reactions. Keeping off of hog meat and fats,
and these eliminated as indicated should be,
we find that it should be a permanent cure."
                                        2392-1

However:

"Know that if there is to be taken, to be sure,
pork, ham, and it is required that there be
taken the acids to digest same--and they are
not taken, this will be hard upon the system.
But if the food values are taken in combinations
and in manners that the system will assimilate
same, this is much preferable." 1259-2

Bacon:

"Not too much of fats. Never hog meat, save
crisp breakfast bacon." 2977-1

"Noons--Preferably vegetables that are well
cooked, preferably WITHOUT fat meats in same.
DO NOT eat hog meat, save the bacon of morning."
                                        1411-2
"Mornings--Citrus fruit with bacon and egg,
and brown toast.
DO NOT eat hog meat, other than the crisp
breakfast bacon." 2959-1

"Q.- Any other advice as to diet?
"A.- As indicated from the slowed circulation,
and the tendencies at times for the acidity,
those things that pertain more to the alkaline-
reacting diet would be the better. Rather
would we give those things that the body should
be warned against, and then most everything
else may be taken if it is taken in moderation,
and when there is the desire! As there is the
desire for food, whether it is the regular
meal time or at others, it would be best for
this body to eat! If it desires to eat this

or that, eat it! but do not mix it with other foods! Beware of hog meats, though, a little crisp bacon may be taken at times." 1016-1

Fowl:

"Plenty of fowl, but prepared in such a way that more of the bone structure itself is used as a part of the diet in its reaction through the system; so that better reaction for the assimilation of calcium through the system is obtained from same.
"Chew chicken necks, then. Chew the bones of the thigh. Also have the marrow of beef, or such, as a part of the diet; eat such foods as the vegetables soups that are right in the beef carrying the marrow of the bone, and the like...and eat the marrow!" 1523-8

"Calcium is now needed, in a manner that it may be assimilated, and gradually take the place of that which has been crystallized in the bursa and portions of the structural body. This we would add in the form which we have indicated as the BEST--the chewing of bones or the ends of bones of the fowl." 849-53

"When fowl is taken choose rather the very small bony pieces rather than what might appear to be the more delicate. Take those that are not supposed to be choice pieces--as the wim-blebit, the back, the neck, the feet. All of these are much preferable and have much more energies for body building." 2948-15

And:

"Keep to those foods that are body-building. When there IS the taxation through the physical exercises have plenty of meats--as fowl, but let these be WELL-DONE. Preferably not the fried foods." 487-22

Chicken:

"Q.- Is it well to eliminate chicken?
"A.- Not necessary to be eliminated from the
system. For there are those vital forces and
balances kept through the system by the acti-
vities of some of these, that are necessary to
be kept in the chemical reaction of the body.
"If chicken would be prepared in certain man-
ners, it would be MOST beneficial; especially
certain portions of same that supply a charac-
ter or an assimilated force of certain elements
that are seldom found in other foods of that
nature--that is, calcium and lime calcium. We
refer to the bony portions, you see, that may
be stewed so that the juice may be chewed from
the same, see? but never fried! (Juice chewed
from the soft BONES, you see.)" 1206-8

"Eat all of the chicken that is possible--
EVERY DAY, but do not fry same or merely roast.
Rather it would be broiled or baked, or cooked
in its own juices inside the oven.
"Then the foods for weight will aid in caring
for the activities through the absorptions and
through the digestive forces." 1560-1

Beef juice:

"Beef juice should be taken regularly--as a
medicine; a teaspoonful four times a day--at
least, but when taken it should be sipped, not
just taken as a gulp." 5374-1

"Also once a day it will be most beneficial
to take beef juice as a tonic; not so much
the beef itself but beef juice; followed with
red wine. Do not mix these, but take both about
the same time. Take about a teaspoonful of the
beef juice, but spend about five minutes in
sipping that much. Then take an ounce of the
red wine, with a whole wheat cracker."
2535-1

"*Q.- What quantity of beef juice to be taken
daily?*
"*A.- At least two tablespoonfuls, but no fat
in same. A tablespoonful is almost equal to a
pound of meat or two pounds of meat a day; and
that's right smart for a man that isn't active.*"

                                            1424-2

Preparation:

"*Pure beef juice, not broth, prepared in this
manner: Take a pound to a pound and a half
(preferably round steak), no fat, no portions
other than the muscle or tendon for strength;
no fatty or skin portions. Dice this into half
inch cubes, as it were, or practically so. Put
same in a glass jar without water in same. Put
the jar into a boiler or container with water
coming about half to three-fourths from the
top of the jar. Put a cloth in the container
to prevent the jar from cracking. Do not seal
the jar tight, but cover the top. Let this boil
(the water, with the jar in same) for three
to four hours.*
"*Then strain off the juice and the refuse may
be pressed somewhat. It will be found that the
meat or flesh itself will be worthless. Place
the juice in a cool place, but do not keep too
long, never longer than three days. Hence the
quantity made up at the time depends upon how
much or how often the body will take this. It
should be taken two or three times a day, but
not more than a tablespoonful at the time--and
this sipped very slowly. Of course, this is to
be seasoned to suit the taste of the body. Well,
too, that whole wheat or Ry-Krisp crackers
be taken with same to make it more palatable.*"

                                            1343-2

Beef:

"*Q.- Should beef be excluded from the diet?*
"*A.- This is not a matter of excluding so much
as to how often and the manner of preparation!*

As we find, it is best that it not be taken too often, though it may be taken at times; that is, once a week, twice a month or the like." 1224-6

"Then, fowl, fish, lamb--and once each week the beef. This should not be hard, but cooked well done, and more of the juice of same taken into the body than the flesh itself." 849-50

"As to meats, we find beef may be taken if it is PREPARED well in its own juices--not so much as a roast, but rather as broiled--but cooking same." 1334-2

"Keep away from meats, especially such as beef; though fish, fowl and lamb may be taken in moderation, but NO FRIED FOODS OF ANY KIND!"
3009-1

SPECIAL FOODS

Almonds:

"And if an almond is taken each day and kept up, you'll never have accumulations of tumors or such conditions through the body. An almond a day is much more in accord with keeping the doctor away, especially certain types of doctors, than apples. For the apple was the fall, not the almond--for the almond blossomed when everything else died. Remember all this is life! 3180-3

"And, just as indicated in other suggestions --those who would eat two or three almonds each day need never fear cancer." 1158-31

"Q.- In what minerals is the body deficient? "A.- As indicated from the type of foods suggested, iron, calcium and phosphorus--these are the ones deficient." 1131-2

"Q.- Please give the foods that would supply these.
"A.- The almond carries more phosphorus and iron in a combination easily assimilated than any other nut."   1131-2

"And know, if ye would take each day, through thy experience, two almonds, ye will never have skin blemishes, ye will never be tempted even in body towards cancer nor towards those things that make blemishes in the body-forces themselves." 1206-13

Jerusalem Artichoke:

"Q.- What about my cravings for sweets.
"A.- This is natural with the indigestion and the lack of proper activity of the pancreas. Eat a Jerusalem artichoke once each week, about the size of an hen egg. Cook this in Patapar paper, preserving all the juices to mix with the bulk of the artichoke. Season to taste. This will also aid in the disorder in the circulation between liver and kidneys, pancreas and kidneys, and will relieve these tensions from the desire for sweets." 3386-2

"As has been indicated for the body, naturally the diet is an important factor in the effect produced upon the assimilating forces of the body itself. Keep away from great quantities of starches. Take those things where the activity in glandular reaction. Especially the Jerusalem artichoke should be a portion of the diet at least once or twice a week." 1482-1

"Instead of using so much insulin; this can be gradually diminished and eventually eliminated entirely if there is used in the diet one Jerusalem artichoke every other day. This should be cooked only in Patapar paper, preserving the juices and mixing with the bulk of

the artichoke, seasoning this to suit the taste. The taking of the insulin is habit forming. The artichoke is never habit forming, never sedative-producing in the body as to cause accumulations of poisons as do sedatives; though it will be necessary to take a sedative when there are the attacks, but take a hypnotic rather than a narcotic--only under the direction, however, of a physician." 4023-1

Salsify (Oyster Plant)

"Also have plenty of those foods such as salsify or oyster plant, especially--that carry those characters of salts that tend to eliminate these hardening centers in the tendons of the body." 2579-1

"Add all of the foods that carry silicon and the salts that may revibrate with the application of the gold to the nerve centers for assimilation; as foods of the tuberous nature of every character--the oyster plant. These should be parts of the foods for the body."
                                        3694-1
"In the matter of the diets, keep those that are body-building. Plenty of oyster plant, once or twice a day, such natures as these would be well as the necessary forces for the better coagulation in the activities of the lymph and the circulatory forces in the blood supply." 560-8

Ginseng:

"Wild ginseng...an essence of the flow of the vitality within the system itself. It is an electrifying of the vital forces themselves."
                                        404-4
"Wild ginseng...increasing their (glands) stability through the life principle as we have in wild ginseng." 839-1

"Wild ginseng will act directly with these combinations (wild cherry bark, sarsaparilla root, etc.) to the activities of the glands of the system; the genitive glands, the lacteal ducts, the lachrymal ducts, the adrenals, the thyroid, all will...with these combinations... make for an activity that is purifying and body-building." 643-1

Potato peelings:

"Add to the diet the Irish potato PEEL, but not the pulp a great deal. It would be better if the nice potatoes are cleansed, peeled and only the PEELINGS cooked and eaten. Throw the other part away, and give it to the chickens, or distribute it in some manner besides eating it." 1904-1

"The skins of the Irish or white potatoes--and that very close to the same--are very good; for the salts in these are well for the body. Even if the potato peels are cooked a long time in water and the juice or soup or broth from same taken; it would be excellent."
2179-1
"Do not use large quantities of potatoes though the peelings of same may be taken at all times--they are strengthening, carrying those influences and forces that are active with the glands of the system." 820-2

Honey, Egg, Lemon:

"To quiet the mucous membrane and to relieve that tendency for irritation, or the cough, we would prepare a combination in these proportions (though a double quantity may be prepared at the time if desired, for it may be kept--and a dose taken two to three times a day):
"Beat the white of an egg until it is very

fluffy. Then, as it has been fluffed, beat
into same a teaspoonful of honey and the juice
of a whole lemon. The dosage would be one to
two to three teaspoonfuls at a time.
"This will work well with the digestive system,
if the fruit juices and vegetable juices are
used--and a little bit later beef juice, and
then the semi liquid foods; as the broth of
chicken, or the broiled chicken or the like
may be then taken.
"Q.- What is the difference in taking into the
system the white of an egg raw, and cooked?
"A.- That depends upon the system, and upon the
manner and with what combinations it is taken.
"For, as we have indicated for this body, it
is not well that the white of the egg be taken,
for it tends to make for an acid reaction. But
when it is beaten very thoroughly first, and
then the honey and the lemon added, the reactions are entirely different; for the properties in same not only react upon the body
through the mucous membranes of the digestive
forces but through the whole of the lymph
circulation, also adding to the system   a
necessary force that is needed in the system
for the assistance of coagulation of the lymph
flow in the creation of the blood cells themselves. It is as the natural reaction to the
yolk of an egg. It isn't that there should be
all acid in any system, not all alkaline; but
it is the reaction of these upon the system
that aids in creating the elements in the
body, see? 808-4

"For any flu or cold, this would be well as
an expectorant and as an eliminant, and to
cause the clearing of hoarseness--made in this
way and manner:
"Take an egg that has not been in the refri-
gerator or cold storage. Take the white of
same. Beat it. Then, to this white of egg, add:
"Juice of one lemon, dropped very slowly into

same. *About a teaspoonful of honey, dropped slowly into same also. About three drops--one at a time--of glycerine.*

"Beat thoroughly together. Of course, it would be worked in together when the glycerine is added.

"Take a teaspoonful every two or three hours.

"We will find this will clear a cold, relieve stress through the throat and the nasal passages, bronchi and larynx, and be most helpful for this body." 845-3

Gelatin:

Gelatin salads were recommended by the readings, since the gelatin acts as a catalyst to increase the natural body's absorption of vitamins. This fact, is unfortunately as little-known as it is significant.

"Do be mindful of the diet, and include often raw vegetables prepared in various ways, not merely as a salad but scraped or grated and combined with gelatin." 3445-1

"In building up the body with the foods, preferably have a great deal of raw vegetables for this body, as lettuce, celery, carrots, watercress. All would be taken raw, with dressing, and oft with gelatin. These should be grated, or cut very fine, or even ground, but do preserve all of the juices with them when these are prepared in this manner with gelatin." 5394-1

"It isn't the vitamin content (of gelatin) but it is its ability to work with the activities of the glands, causing the glands to take from that which is absorbed or digested, the vitamins that would not be active in the body if there is or were not sufficient gelatin in the body. See, these may be mixed with any chemical that which make the rest of the system sus-

ceptible or able to call from the system that
which is beeded. It becomes, then, "sensitive"
to conditions. Without it there is not that
sensitivity to vitamins." 849-75

"Also every day we would take gelatin as an
aid to the quick pick-up for energy, aiding the
system--from the assimilation of this with
the chemical changes in the body--in creating
those activities through the assimilating and
glandular force for the energies that create
corpuscle tissue in body. This we would take
about a third of a teaspoonful stirred in a
glass of COLD water each day. If this is taken
around two or three o'clock in the afternoon,
it will aid the more." 2737-1

DIET

"As to the diet, this should carry a great
deal of the salts of vegetables AND fruits--
rather than meats. Never any fried foods at
any time. The vegetables should be cooked in
their OWN juices--that is, in Patapar paper.
The juices that come from same shall be well
mixed with the vegetables themselves, so that
the body gets the benefit of those; such as
cabbage with their salts as come from same--
after being well washed and cooked in the
Patapar paper, but DO NOT put meat or anything
of the kind in same. Season only with a little
butter and sufficient salt or pepper to satisfy
appetite or to be palatable to the taste of
the body." 1659-1

"Q.- Please explain the reaction of foods upon
my system.
"A.- It's just been given! Those that require
the bodily foods--there are foods that require
(as meats) acids for their proper fermentation
while most of the leafy nature, require more
of the slow combination of the lacteals' reac-

tion or the greater quantity of the combination
of acid and alkaline. Then if foods are taken
in quantities that require an alkaline for
their digestion and an acid is in the system
--this produces improper fermentation.If foods
are taken where acid is necessary and it is
not produced by the system, or not taken into
the system in synthetic state, then these
produce the disturbances, see? See how the
combinations of these, then, make for the
necessity of watching, experimenting as it
were with that which is good today and may be
bad tomorrow. For what would be poison for
someone, to another may be a cure. This is
true in every physical organism. And unless
the balances are being cared for properly,
they produce disturbances." 1259-2

"Q.- Please suggest things to be stressed and
things to be avoided in the diet.
"A.- Avoid too much combinations of starches.
Do not take a combination of potatoes, meat,
white bread, macaroni or macaroni and cheese,
at the same meal; not two of these at any one
meal, though they each may be taken separately
at other times, or as a lunch or a part of a
separate meal. Avoid raw meats, or rare meats
that are not well cooked. Not too much ever
of hog meat. Have plenty of vegetables, and
especially one meal each day should include
some raw or uncooked vegetables. But here,
too, combinations must be kept in line. Don't
take onions and radishes at the same meal with
celery and lettuce, though either of these may
be taken at different times, see." 2732-1

"Those foods, now, that are the body-building;
as starches and proteins, if these are taken
without other food values that make for the
combinations that produce distress or disorder;
that is, not quantities of starches and proteins combined, you see, but these taken one

*at one meal and one at another will be most
helpful. As potatoes, whether white or the
yam activity with butter, should not be taken
with fats or meats; but using these as a portion of one meal with fruits or vegetables is
well. When meats are taken, use mutton, fowl
or the like, and do not have heavy starches
with same--but preferably fruits or vegetables." 805-2*

*"The DIET--this must be, as the rest, CONSIS-
TENTLY, PERSISTENTLY followed.
"Take more of the vegetable forces that are
life giving in their assimilation through the
body; CARROTS etc. These should be combined
to make the greater part of one meal each day;
or they may be taken with EACH meal if it is
the more preferable. They MUST BE TAKEN, if
there will be better recuperative forces, or
the supplying to the system of properties and
energies that are to be the real HEALING forces.
"For here alone (in the diet) will there be
the coming of curative or healing powers. All
the rest are for the PREPARATIONS of the body
for the USAGE of energies in food values,
which may be had from those foods indicated
to be supplied." 849-47*

*"In the matter of diets: Here we need body-
building foods but those that tend to be more
alkaline-producing than acid. For the natural
inclinations of disturbed conditions in a body
are to produce acidity through the blood
stream. Hence we need to revivify same by the
use of much of those that produce more of the
enzymes, more of the hormones for the blood
supply; yet not overburdening the body with
those unless the balance in the vitamin forces
is carried.
"Hence as we will find, not heavy foods or
fried foods ever, nor combinations where there
are quantities of starches or quantities of*

starches with sweets taken at the same time.
But fish, fowl or lamb preferably as the meats."
                                           1302-1
"Not such a diet as to be contrary to natural
laws, but that which is in keeping with the
manner in which the body exerts itself--so
that there may be brought the better resuscitating influences and forces.
"Upon the natural things, then, that replenish and supply energies--as in these; not as
the only things eaten, but this as an outline
for the activities of the body to preserve and
maintain a balance." 1662-1

As a practical illustration, reading # 3823-3
describes briefly the daily dietary regimen as is
followed by the Cayce health enthusiast:

"As an outline, we would give:
"Mornings (this is not all to be taken, but
as an outline)--citrus fruits juices. When
orange juice is taken add lime or lemon juice
to same; four parts orange to one part lime or
lemon. When other citrus fruits are taken, as
pineapple or grapefruit, they may be taken as
they are from the fresh fruit. A little salt
added to same is preferable...
"Whole wheat bread, toasted, browned, with
butter. Coddled egg, only the yolk of same. A
small piece of very crisp bacon if so desired.
Any or all of these may be taken.
"But when cereals are taken, do not have citrus
fruits at the same meal...Such a combination
produces just what we are trying to prevent
in the system!
"When cereals are used, have either cracked
wheat or whole wheat, or a combination of
barley and wheat--as in Maltex, if these are
desired, or Puffed Wheat, or Puffed Rice, or
Puffed Corn--any of these. And these may be
taken with certain characters of fresh fruits;
as berries of any nature, even strawberries

*if so desired. (No, they won't cause any of
the rash if they are taken properly!), or
peaches. The sugar used should only be saccharin or honey. A cereal drink may be had if
so desired.*

*"Noons--only raw fresh vegetables. All of these
may be combined, but grate them--don't eat
them so that they would make for that combination which often comes with not the proper
mastication. Each time you take a mouthful,
even if it's water, it should be chewed at
least four to twenty times; whether it's water
or bread or a carrot, onion, cabbage, or what!
Each should be chewed so that there is the
mastication, and that there is the opportunity
for the flow of the gastric forces from the
salivary glands well mixed with same. Then we
will find that these will make for bettered
conditions.*

*"Evenings--vegetables that are cooked in their
own juices, not combined with others--each
cooked alone, then combined together afterward
if so desired by the body, see? These may
include any of the leafy vegetables or any of
bulbular ones, cook them in their own juices!
There may be taken the meats, if so desired by
the body, or there may be added the proteins
that come from the combination of other vegetables or combination of vegetable forces in
the forms of certain character of pulse or of
grains." 3823-3*

Once again:

*"Mornings--citrus fruits, cereals or fruits,
but do not mix citrus fruits and cereals,
though stewed fruits may be taken; or citrus
fruits, and a little later rice cakes, or
buckwheat or Graham cakes, with honey in the
honeycomb, with milk or the like, and preferably the raw milk, if certified milk!*

"Noons--rather vegetables juices than meat

juices, with raw vegetables as a salad or the
like.

"Evenings--vegetables, with such as carrots,
peas, salsify, red cabbage, yams or white
potatoes--these the smaller variety, with the
jackets the better; using as the finishing,
or desert, those of blancmange or jello, or
jellies, with fruits--as peaches, apricots,
fresh pineapple or the like. These as we find
with the occasional sufficient meats for
strength, would bring a well-balanced diet.
"Occasionally we would add those of the blood
building, once or twice a week. The pig knuck-
les, tripe and calves liver or those of the
brains and the like." 275-24

INOCULATIONS

"Keep closer to the alkaline diets; using
fruits, berries, vegetables particularly that
carry iron, silicon, phosphorus and the like
--and those as we have indicated.
"Q.- Are inoculations against contagious diseases necessary for me before sailing in
September?
"A.- As we find, only where the requirements
are such as to demand same would this be
adhered to at all. So far as the body-physical
conditions is concerned, the adherence to the
use of carrots every day as a meal or as a
portion of the meal will insure against any
contagious infectious forces with which the
body may be in contact.
"Q.- Can immunization against them be set up
in any other manner than by inoculation?
"A.- As indicated, if alkalinity is maintained
in the system--especially with carrots, these
in the blood supply will maintain such a condition as to immunize a person." 480-19

"Q.- Were hayfever shots in any way responsible
for this trouble?

*"A.- Any shots are responsible for most any-
thing! Yes, they are a part of the disorders."*
                                    3629-1
"Q.- Would sulfa drugs help the strep condition?
"A.- And make you worse in other conditions?
Yes." 3287-2

*"There is no infection, as indicated, of tu-
bercular inflammation. But (there are) the
adhesions, and these were produced by the
after-effects of the sulfa drug. While this
drug, to be sure, destroyed those inflammations
of the natures (described) in the lobe of the
lung itself, yet it is like saying the operation
is successful but the patient died. So it (the
sulfa), is successful in eliminating the character of inflammation or the bug which was
infectious; But the adhesions in the same (lung
area) are causing the greater trouble."*
                                    294-98

At present the trend of medical science, is
undoubtedly toward the injections of serum, antitoxin,
and vaccine treatment. Recently all medical research
tends that way. Every few days we see in local daily
papers reports of some new serums and antitoxins for
which they claim the ability to cure and for creating
immunity to certain diseases.

Suppose the research and practice of medical
science continue along these lines and are generally
accepted or, as the medical associations would have
it, forced upon the public by law. What would be the
results? Before a child reached adolescence, it would
have been injected into its blood stream numerous
vaccines, serums, and antitoxins of questionable characters of no mean consequence.

If doctors were to have their way, the blood of
the adult would be a mixture of dozens of filthy
bacterial extracts, disease taints, and destructive
drug poisons. The tonsils and adenoids, the appendix
vermiformis, and probably a few other parts of the
human anatomy would be extirpated in early youth under
the compulsion of the Health Departments in various

parts of the country.

What is more rational and sensible; the endeavor to produce immunity to disease by making the human body the breeding ground for all sorts of anti-bacterial and anti-poisons, or to create natural immunity by building up the blood on a normal basis, purifying the body of morbid matter and poisons, correcting mechanical lesions, and by cultivating the right mental attitude? Which one of these methods is more likely to be disease-building and which health-building?

Just imagine what human blood will be like in coming generations if this artificial contaminations with all sorts of disease taints and drug poisons is to be forced upon innocent people.

Also:

> "There is so easily an overstressing upon milk, by many; for there are many products much more healthful than milk. So few milks are free from tubercle: so few are free from those influences that cause a great deal more irritation than help--unless irradiated or dried milk is used. These as a whole are much more healthful to most individuals than raw milk." 480-22

This treatise on dietetics is not in any manner complete but enough is presented here that a general view may be obtained of this vast subject.

CHAPTER SEVENTEEN

FASTING

Next in importance to building up the blood on a natural basis is the elimination of waste, morbid matter, and poisons from the system. This depends to a large extent upon the right (natural) diet; but it must be promoted by the different methods of eliminative treatment: fasting, hydrotherapy, massage, physical exercise, air and sun baths, and in the way of medicinal treatment, by homeopathic and herbal remedies.

Foremost among the methods of purification stands fasting, which in some respects, has become very popular and is regarded by many people as a panacea for all human ailments. However, it is a two-edged sword. According to circumstances, it may do a great deal of good or a great deal of harm.

It is claimed that disease is a "unit," that it consists of, accumulation of waste and morbid matter in the system. Since olden times, many "naturalist," have claimed that fasting offers the best and the quickest means for eliminating systemic poisonous wastes.

To "fast it out" seems simple and plausible, but it does not always prove to be successful in practice. Fasting enthusiasts forget that the elimination of waste and morbid matter from the system is more of a chemical than a mechanical process. They also overlook the fact that in many cases of lowered vitality and weakened powers of resistance, diseases precede and make possible the accumulation of morbid matter in the organism.

If the encumbrances consists merely of superflous flesh, or of fat or of accumulated waste materials, fasting may be sufficient to break up the accumulation and to eliminate the impurities that are therefore clogging the blood and tissues of the body.

If, however, the distress has its origin in other than mechanical causes, or if it be due to a weakened, negative constitution and lowered powers of resistance, fasting may aggravate the abnormal conditions instead of improving them.

We hear frequently of long fasts, as a form of protest, extending over days and weeks, undertaken recklessly without the prescription and guidance of a competent dietetic advisor, without proper preparation of the system and the right subsequent treatment. Many a good constitution has thus been permanently injured and absolutely wrecked.

WHEN FASTING IS INDICATED

Persons of sanguine, vital temperament, with the animal qualities strongly developed, enslaved by bad habits and evil passions, will be greatly benefited by occasional short fasts. In such cases the experience affords a fine drill in self-discipline, strenghtening of self-control, and conquest of the lower appetites.

Vigorous fleshy people, positive physically and mentally, especially those who do not take sufficient physical exercise, should take frequent fast of one, two, or three days duration for the reduction of super-fluous flesh and fat, and for the elimination of systematic waste and other morbid matter. Such people should never eat more than two meals a day, and many get along best on only one meal.

However, different temperaments and constitutions require different treatment and management.

People of a nervous and emotional temperament, especially those who are below normal in weight and physically and mentally negative, may be seriously and permanently injured by fasting. They should never fast except in acute diseases and during eliminative healing crises, when nature calls for the fast as a means of cure.

People of this type are usually thin, with weak and flabby muscles. Their vital activities are at a low ebb and their magnetic envelope (the aura) are wasted and attenuated like their physical bodies. The red aura, which is created by the action of the purely animal functions and forces is more or less deficient or entirely lacking. Such people have the tendency to become abnormally sensitive to conditions in the magnetic field (the astral plane).

Next to the hypnotic or mediumistic process, there is nothing that induces abnormal psychism so quickly as fasting. During a prolonged fast, the purely animal functions of digestion, assimilation, and elimination are almost completely at a standstill. This repression of the physical functions causes and increases the psychic functions and may produce intense emotionalism and abnormal activity of the senses of the spiritual body. The individual thus becoming abnormally clairvoyant, clairaudient, and otherwise sensitive to conditions on the spiritual plane of life.

This explains the spiritual exaltation and the visions of heavenly scenes and beings or the fights with demons which are frequently, indeed uniformly, reported by hermits, ascetics, saints, etc.

Fasting facilitates hypnotic control of the sensitive by positive intelligences, either on the physical, or on the spiritual plane of being. In one case we speak of hypnotism, in the other, of mediumship, obsession, or possession. These conditions are usually diagnosed by the regular practitioner as nervousness, nervous prostration, hysteria, double personality, paranoia, delusional insanity, mania, etc.

For destructive effects of fasting are intensified by solitude, grief, worry, introspection, physical exaltation, or any other form of depressive and or destructive mental or emotional activity.

Spirit "control" often force their subjects to abstain from food altogether, thus rendering them still more negative and submissive. Psychic patients, when controlled or obsessed, will frequently not eat unless they are forced or fed like an infant. When asked why they do not want to eat, these patients reply: "I must not. They will not let me." When we say: "Who?" the answer is: "These people. Don't you see them?" pointing to a void, and becoming impatient when told that no one is there. The regular school says "delusion"; we call it abnormal clairvoyance. Psychiatry calls it, Anorexia Nervosa.

The term Anorexia (loss of appetite) Nervosa (due to nerves) is a severe psychological problem according to psychiatrists. Victims of this disease, almost always young women, begin losing weight and then cannot stop. In the pursuit of a seemingly elusive thinness, anorexics starve themselves, sometimes to death. And recent studies do note that approximately one out of every 100 adolescent girls suffers from anorexia.

Although the disease has been discussed in medical circles for nearly three centuries, its underlying, unknown causes and proper treatment are still being debated. Most doctors, however, are agreeable on the symptoms of anorexia.

We are a diet conscious society, and excessive dieting is considered acceptable. People are caught up in thinking that "thinner is better," but in the case of the anorexic victim, thinner can be deadly.

To place persons of the negative, sensitive type on prolonged fast and thus to expose them to the danger just described, is little short of criminal, if not. Such patients need an abundance of the most positive animal and vegetable foods in order to build up and strengthen their physical bodies and their magnetic envelopes, which form the dividing and protecting wall between the terrestrial plane and the spiritual plane.

A negative vegetarian diet, consisting almost of fruits, nuts, cereals, and pulses, but deficient in animal foods (meat, dairy products, eggs, honey) and in the vegetables growing in or near the ground, may result in conditions similar to those which accompany prolonged fasting.

Some animal foods are thereby elaborated under the influence of a higher life-element than those controlling the vegetable kingdom, and foods derived from the animal kingdom are necessary to develop and stimulate the positive qualities of man.

Interestingly enough, Cayce gave the following in answer to a question regarding this matter.

"Q.- Is there any combinations of foods that could be truthfully called Brain Foods, Nerve

Foods, Muscles Foods?
"A.- Those that are body-building; those that
are nerve-building and those that supply
certain elements. For as indicated, those
foods suggested are to be taken by the body.
Fish, fowl and lamb are those that supply
elements needed for brain, muscle and nerve-
building." 4008-1

In the case of the psychic who is already deficient
in the physical (animal), and over-developed in the
spiritual qualities, it is especially necessary, in
order to restore and maintain the lost equilibrium, to
build up in him the animal qualities needed for brain,
muscle and nerve elements.

HOW TO FAST

Before, during, and after a therapeutic fast,
everything must be done to keep the eliminations active,
in order to prevent the re-absorption of the toxins
that are being stirred up and liberated.

Fasting involves rapid breaking-down of the tissues. This creates great quantities of worn-out cell
materials and other morbid substances. Unless these
poison producing accumulations are promptly eliminated
they will be reabsorbed into the system and cause
auto-intoxication.

To prevent this, bowels, kidneys, and skin must
be kept in an active condition. The diet, for several
days before and after a fast, should consist largely
of uncooked fruits and vegetables, and the different
methods of natural stimulative treatment should be
systematically applied.

During a fast, every bit of vitality must be
economized; therefore the passive treatments are to be
preferred to active exercises, though a certain amount
of exercise (especially walking) daily out in the open
air, accompanied with deep breathing, should not ever
be neglected.

While fasting, intestinal evacuation will usually
cease, especially where there is a natural tendency to

sluggishness of the bowels. Injections are therefore in order and during prolonged fasts may be taken every few days.

In prolonged fasts we are talking of fasts that last from one to four weeks, while short fasts being those of one, two, or three days duration. The latter fasts are the most beneficial.

Moderate drinking is beneficial during a fast as well as at other times; but excessive consumption of water, the so-called "flushing of the system," is very injurious. Under ordinary conditions from five to eight glasses of water a day are probably sufficient; the quantity consumed must be regulated, of course, by the desire of the one that is fasting.

Those who are fasting should mix their drinking water with the juice of acid fruits, preferably lemon or orange. These juices act as eliminators, and also are fine natural antiseptics. The readings recommend fruit juices as a great revitalizer.

> *"Let the diet be only fruit juices, principally lemons. A little orange juice may be taken, but mix it rather with the lemon. And the other periods of diet would consist of vegetable juices." 555-4*

This brings to the fore a number of intriguing concepts given by Edgar Cayce for a complete fast. The variations, of course, depends on what is to be gained or overcome by the body.

Juice diets:

> *"With the cold and congestion in the present, almost an entire liquid diet would be the better. Grapefruit juice, taken with a little salt rather than sugar in same. They may be taken two or three times a day, provided the body can be induced to take same." 738-2*

> *"Let the diet be only fruit juices, principally grapefruit. And the other periods of*

diet would consist of vegetable juices."

555-4

"Then in meeting the needs in the present we would find that we would first give an outline to prepare the body; for later--as we will find--it will be necessary to change the order of these things that would be applied for the corrections to be permanent; for the effects, as well as some portion of the causes, must be attended to first. First, then:

"For at least three to five days, let the diet be only grapefruit juice and grapes.

"Q.- Should the grapefruit juice and grapes be taken at the same time?

"A.- No! One at one time, one at the other. But eat quantities of grapes--whether two, three, four, five or ten pounds, even!"133-3

Orange diet:

"There may be the use of citrus fruit juices in quantities: but this would necessitate, then, that there be not too great an activity, and that nothing else be taken but the citrus fruit for five days. This would include only oranges, or oranges with lemons--no other foods--for five days. Just how many? As many as the body wants to take!

"On the evening of the last day of such a diet --take half a teacup of olive oil. This would cleanse the system from the impurities, preventing the inclinations for gas formation and for this regurgitation that is taking place in the lower portion of the duodenum."

1713-21

"Q.- What should the body do to overcome constipation?

"A.- We would first, for at least three to five days, beginning now, be on a diet chiefly of oranges, see? Then after three days (for we will find this will tend to cleanse the alimentary canal, especially the colon), we would begin

with those of the filling or heavy diet.
"Q.- How many oranges should be taken each day?
"A.- About a dozen." 1713-17

"As to the diet after the first cleansing with
the apples--we would have plenty of oranges."
                                              2423-1

Apple diet:

"As to apples--as we have indicated oft-these
are not best for most people, except under
conditions where they are advisable to be taken
ALONE as a diet for the eliminations, or where
certain characters of apples or their products
are taken. Hence for this body, these we will
leave off." 1206-8

"If there is the desire on the part of the
body to test self for tape worms, live for
three days on raw apples only! Then take about
half a teacup of olive oil, or half a glass of
olive oil. And this should remove fecal matter
that hasn't been removed for some time! But
it will certainly indicate there is no tape
worm!" 567-7

"It would be well for this body, even after
this, to have a three-day apple diet, even in
its weakened condition we need to clear the
system. For this will get rid of the tendencies
for neuritic conditions in the joints of the
body. Also take the olive oil after the three
day diet. But don't go without the apples--eat
them--all you can--at least five or six apples
each day. Chew them up, scrape them well. Drink
plenty of water, and follow the three-day diet
with the big dose of olive oil." 1409-9

Buttermilk and banana diet:

"While there are the indications of the ten-
dency for the humor or the effluvia in the

*blood to cause greater disturbances (because
of overtaxation of the body physically), we
find that these will respond to the adherence
to those suggestions as we have indicated--
either the yeast, as an eliminant, or the
buttermilk and bananas as a builder-up AND a
tearer-down in some direction (for these work
with the effluvia of the intestinal system for
better eliminations).*
*"Q.- Should I go on the three-day diet of
buttermilk and bananas?*
*"A.- Two days should be sufficient, or three
days if so desired." 538-60*

*"Q.- Would it be better to use bananas or some
other fruit for the diet?*
*"A.- Use the bananas and the buttermilk. Then
continue, of course, with a little of the
buttermilk; and don't eat too heavily of ANY
foods that are too acid.*
*"Q.-Should I continue the yeast tablets during
the three day diet?*
*"A.- If necessary for the better elimination,
continue with same throughout the period of
the diet." 538-58*

Grape diet:

*"We would be mindful that the diet is that
which is easily assimilated. Not too great
quantities of starch foods, but sufficient to
aid in creating the proper balance in those
periods of assimilation necessary for proper
fermentation. We would not have too great
quantities of sugar. Or the body may, under
the existent circumstances, go on an entire
grape diet--see, entire grape diet, for at
least three day periods; then to the regular
normal diet that has been indicated. Quantities
of grapes! And should there appear any disturbance in the stomach and duodenum through
these periods, make a poultice of the grape*

hull and pulp--between cloths--and apply over those areas; or over the abdomen and liver area you see. Make this about an inch and a half thick--that large quantity, you see, all over. Plenty of water, but just grapes for three days--quantities all that the body can eat."
                                                    757-6

"Some days, for at least three of four days, eat only GRAPES! Not with the seed, to be sure, but preferably those of the purple variety; not the larger but those that are good and NOT those that have been shipped or kept too long."
                                                    1703-1

"We find it would be helpful to have three or four days each month when only grapes would be used as the diet. And during those three to four days we would apply the grape poultices across all of the abdomen itself." 683-3

While fasting, the right emotional attitude and purpose is all important. Unless you can do it with perfect equanimity, without fear or misgiving, do not fast at all. Destructive mental conditions may more than offset the beneficial effects of the fast.

To recapitulate: never undertake a prolonged fast unless you have been properly prepared by natural diet and treatment, and never without the guidance of a competent advisor.

However, fasting should not begin until the right physiological and psychological moment has arrived, until the feel of the fast is indicated. And when the organism, or rather the individual cell, is ready to begin the work of elimination, then assimilation should cease for the time being, because it interferes with the excretory processes going on in the system.

To fast before the system is ready for it, means mineral-salts starvation and defective eliminations.

Given a vigorous positive constitution, encumbered with too much flesh and with a tendency to chronic constipation, rheumatism, gout, apoplexy, and other diseases due to food-poisoning, a fast may be indicated from the beginning. But it is different with persons of the weak, negative type.

Ordinarily, the organism resembles a huge sponge, which absorbs all the elements of nutrition from the digestive tract. During a fast the process is reversed, the sponge being squeezed gives off the impurities contained within it.

However, this is a purely mechanical process and deals only with the mechanical aspect of disease, with the presence of waste matter in the system. It does not take into consideration the chemical aspect of disease.

We have learned that most of the morbid matter in the system has its origin in the acid waste products of starchy and protein digestion.

In rheumatism and gout, the colloid (glue-like) and earthy deposits collect in the joints and muscular tissues; in arteriolesis, in the arteries and veins, in paralysis, epilepsy, and kindred disease, in brain and nerve tissues.

The accumulation of these waste products is due, in turn to a deficiency in the system of the alkaline, acid-burning and acid-eliminating mineral elements. As a matter of fact, almost every form of disease is characterized by a lack of these organic mineral salts in the blood and tissues.

Stones, gravel, etc., grow in acid blood only, and must be dissolved and eliminated by rendering the blood alkaline. This is accomplished by the absorption of the alkaline salts, contained most abundantly in the juicy fruits, the leafy and juicy vegetables, the hulls of cereal, as well as in milk.

How, then, are these all-important solvents and eliminators to be supplied to the organism by total abstinence from foods.

Prolonged fasting undoubtedly lowers the person's vitality and his powers of resistance to disease. But natural elimination of waste products and systemic poisons depends upon increased vitality and activity of the organism and its individual cells.

For these reasons we find, in most cases, that proper adjustment of the diet, both as to quality and quantity, together with the different forms of natural

corrective and stimulative treatment must precede
the fasting.

The great majority of chronic patients have become
"chronic" because their skin, kidneys, intestines, and
other organs of elimination are in a sluggish, atrophied
condition. As a result, their systems are overloaded
with morbid matter.

Moreover, during the fast the system has to live
on its own tissues, which are being broken down rapidly.
This results in the production and liberation of additional large quantities of morbid matter and poisons,
which must be promptly eliminated so as to prevent
their re-absorbtion.

However, the atrophic condition of the organs of
elimination makes this impossible, and there are not
enough alkaline mineral elements to neutralize the
destructive acids. Therefore, the impurities remain
and accumulate in the system and may cause serious
aggravations and complications.

Is it not wiser first of all to build up the blood
on a normal basis by natural diet, and to put the organs
of elimination in good working order by the natural
methods of treatment before fasting is undertaken?
This is indeed, the only, rational procedure, and will
always be followed by the best possible results

When, under the influence of a rational diet, the
blood has regained its normal composition, when mechanical obstructions to the free flow of blood and nerve
currents have been removed by osteopathic treatment,
when skin, kidney, bowels, nerves and nerve centers,
in fact, every cell in the body has been stimulated
into vigorous activity by the various methods, of
natural treatment, then the cells themselves begin to
eliminate their own morbid encumbrances. As the waste
materials are carried in the blood stream to the organs
of elimination they excite them to acute reactions in
the form of diarrheas, catarrhal discharges, fevers,
inflammations, skin eruptions, boils, abscesses, etc.

Now the sponge is being squeezed and cleansed of
its impurities in a natural manner. The mucous membrane
of the stomach and bowels are called upon to assist
in the work of house-cleaning; hence the coated tongue,

lack of appetite, digestive disturbances, flatulence, nausea, biliousness, sour stomach, fermentation, and occasional vomiting and purging.

These digestive disturbances are always accompanied by mental depression, "the blues," homesickness, irritability, fear, hopelessness, etc.

With the advent of these cleansing and healing crises the physiological and psychological moment for fasting has arrived. All the processes of digestion are at a standstill. The entire organism is eliminating and will eventually clear itself of all toxins.

We have learned that these healing crises usually arrive during the sixth week of natural treatment.

To take food now would mean to force assimilation and thereby stop elimination and perchance to interfere with or to check a beneficial healing crisis.

Therefore, it is absolutely essential to stop eating as soon as any form of acute elimination makes its appearance, and not take any food except acid fruits juices diluted with water until all signs of acute eliminative activity has subsided, whether this requires a few days or a few weeks or a few months.

To promote the eliminations, water in the amount of six to eight glasses daily is a requisite to achieve a normal balance in the body.

> "...there should be more water taken into the system in a more consistent manner, so that the system, especially in the hepatics and kidneys, may function more normally, thus producing the correct manner for elimination of drosses in the system, for, as we see, there are many channels of elimination from the system. For this reason, each channel should be kept in that equilibrium or in that balance wherein the condition is not brought to an accentuated condition in any one of the eliminating functioning conditions; not overtaxing the lungs, not overtaxing the kidneys, not overtaxing the liver, not overtaxing the respiratory system, but all kept in that equal manner...

*"The lack of this water in the system creates,
then, the excess of those eliminations that
should normally be cleansed through alimentary
canal and through the kidneys, back to the
capillary circulation....(This brings about,
at times,) congestion and weakened condition."*
                                                    257-11

Therefore:

*"In the diet--do live mostly, for a while, on
watermelon, carrots, beets almost daily. The
watermelon is for the activity of the liver
and kidney.*
*"Most of all, pray. Let the mental attitude be
considered first and foremost. Do not promise
thyself, nor thy God, nor thy neighbor that
you do not fulfill." 3121-1*

Consider:

*"Fasting means what the Master gave: laying
aside our own concept of HOW or WHAT should
be done at any period and letting the SPIRIT
guide. Get the TRUTH of fasting!*
*"To be sure, overindulgence in bodily appetites
brings shame to self, as overindulgences in
anything. But TRUE fasting is casting out of
self any thought of what WE would have done
and becoming CHANNELS for what HE, the LORD,
would have done in the earth through us."*
                                                    295-2

CHAPTER EIGHTEEN

CORRECT BREATHING

The lungs are to the body what the bellows are to the fires of the forge. The more regularly and vigorously the air is forced through the bellows and through the lungs, the livelier is the burn of the flame in the smithy and the fires of life in the body.

Practice deep, regular breathing systematically for one week, and you will be surprised at the results. You will feel like a different person, and your working capacity, born physically and mentally, will also be immensely increased.

A plentiful supply of fresh air is more necessary in a way than food and drink. We can live without food for weeks, without water for days, but without air only a few minutes.

With every inhalation, air is sucked in through the windpipe or trachea, which terminates in two tubes called bronchi, one leading to the right lung, one to the left. The air is then distributed over the lungs through a network of minute tubes, to the air cells, which are separated only by a thin membrane from the equally fine and minute blood vessels forming another network of tubes.

The oxygen contained in the inhaled air passes freely through these membranes, is absorbed by the blood, carried to the heart, and thence through the arteries and their branches to the different organs and tissues of the body, fanning the fires of life into brighter flames all along its course, and burning up the waste products and poisons that have accumulated during the vital processes of digestion, assimilation, and elimination.

After the blood has unloaded its supply of oxygen, it takes up the carbonic acid gas which is produced during the oxidation and combustion of waste matter, and carries it to the lungs, where the poisonous gases

are transferred to the air cells and expelled with
the exhaled breath. This return trip of the blood to
the lungs is made through another set of blood vessels, the veins, and the blood, dark with the sewage
of the system, is now called "venous" blood.

In the lungs the venous blood discharges its
freight of excrementitious poisons and gases, and by
coming in contact with fresh air and a new supply of
oxygen, it it once again transferred into bright, red
"arterial" blood, pregnant with oxygen and ozone, the
life-sustaining element of the atmosphere.

This explains why normal, deep, regular breathing
is all-important to sustain life and as a means of
cure. By proper breathing, which exercises and develops
every part of the lungs, the capacity of the air cells
is increased. This, as we have learned, means also an
increased supply of life-sustaining and health-promo-
ting oxygen to the tissues of the body.

However:

Very few people breathe correctly. Some, woman
especially with tight skirt-bands and corset-like un-
dergarments pressing upon their vital organs, use only
the upper part of their lungs. Others, breathe only
with the lower part and with the diaphram, leaving the
upper structures of the lungs inactive and collapsed.

In those parts of the lungs that are not used,
slimy secretions accumulate, irritating the air cells
and other tissues, which become inflammed and therefore
begins to decay. Thus a luxuriant soil is prepared for
the tubercle bacillus, the pneumococcus, and other
disease-producing bacilli and germs such as colds.

This habit of shallow breathing, which does not
allow the lungs to be thoroughly permeated with fresh
air, accounts in a measure for the fact that one-third
of all deaths results from disease of the lungs. For
every individual perishing from food starvation, many
thousands are dying from oxygen starvation.

Lung-culture is more important than any other
branches of learning and training which requires more
time than a greater outlay of time, money, and effort.

All in all, the regimen of the breathing exercises play an important part in the health of individuals.

The effectiveness of breathing exercises and of all other kinds of corrective movements depends upon the mental attitude during the time of practice. Each motion should be accompanied by the conscious effort to make it produce a certain result. Much more can be accomplished with mental concentration, by keeping the mind on what one is doing, rather than by performing the exercises in an aimless and indifferent way.

"To be sure, in the present period, present development, present conditions that exist, must be gone at gently; but be persistent morning and evening, working at it, still not letting it become rote, but purposeful."

681-2

Keep in the open air as much as possible, and at all events sleep with the windows open.

"The entity should keep close to all of those things that have to do with outdoor activities, for it is the best way to keep yourself young --to stay close to nature, close to those activities in every form of exercise that... Breathe it into thine own soul, as you would a sunset or a morning sun rising. And see that sometimes--it's as pretty as the sunset!"

3374-1

"Walk in the open early of mornings. This brings better activity of oxygen and ozone as to keep the balance in the blood flow through lungs, heart, liver, kidneys. These are the sources from which either the pressure or repression causes disturbances." 2533-6

"Well that the body take each day a certain amount of exercise, or as much as possible in the open. Walking is the best exercise, but this --though--in the OPEN when at all practical."

1530-2

If your occupation is sedentary, take all the opportunities for walking out of doors that present themselves. When walking, breathe regularly and deeply, filling the lungs to their fullest capacity and also expelling as much air as possible at each exhalation. This applies to all breathing exercises as well.

Do not breathe through the mouth. Nature intends, that the outer air shall reach the lungs by way of the nose, whose membranes are lined with fine hairs in order to "sift" out the air and to prevent foreign particles, dust and dirt, from penetrating and irritating the mucous linings of the air tract and entering the delicate structures of the lungs. Also, the air is warmed before it reaches the lungs by its passage through the nose.

Let the exhalations take about double the time of the inhalations. This will be further explained in connection with rhythmical breathing.

Do not hold the breath between inhalations. Though recommended frequently by teachers of certain methods of breath-culture, this practice is more harmful than beneficial. However an alternate nostril breathing is recommended as being very energizing.

> "Of morning, and upon arising especially (and don't sleep too late!)--and before dressing so that the clothing is loose or the fewer the better--standing erect before an open window, breathe deeply; gradually raising hands ABOVE the head, and then with the circular motion of the body from the hips bend forward; breathing IN (and through the nostrils) as the body rises on its toes--breathing very deep; EXHALING SUDDENLY through the MOUTH, NOT through the (NOSE) nasal passages. Take these (exercises) for 5 or 6 minutes. Then as these progress, gradually CLOSE one of the nostrils (even if it's necessary to use the hand--but if it is closed with the left hand, raise the right hand; and when closing the right nostril with the right hand, then raise the left hand) AS the breathing IN is accomplished." 1523-2

Of great importance is that the position assumed habitually by the body not only while standing and

walking but also when exercising. Carelessness in this
respect is not only unpleasant to the beholder, but its
consequences are far-reaching in their effects upon
the health and well-being of the organism.

On the other hand, a good carriage of the body
aids in the development of muscles and tissues generally, and in the proper functioning of cells and
organs in particular. With the weight of the body
thrown upon the balls of the feet and the center of
gravity well focused, the abdominal organs will stay
in place and there will be no strain upon the ligaments
that support them.

In assuming the proper standing position, stand
with your back to the wall, touching it with heels,
buttocks, shoulders, and head. Now bend the head backward and push the shoulders forward and away from the
wall, still touching the wall with buttocks and heels.
Straighten the head, keeping the shoulders in the
forward position. Now walk away from the wall and endeavor to maintain this position while taking the breathing
exercises and practicing the various arm movements.

Take this position as often as possible during the
day, and try to maintain it while you go about your
different tasks that must be performed while standing.
Gradually this position will become second nature,
and you will assume and maintain it without effort.

When the body is in this position, the viscera
are in their normal place. This aids the indigestion
materially and benefits indirectly the entire body as
a functional organism.

Persistent practice of the above will correct
protuding abdomen and other defects due to faulty
position and carriage of the body.

The following breathing exercises are intended
especially to develop greater lung-capacity and to
assist in forming the habit of breathing properly at
all times. The different movements should be repeated
from three to six times, according to endurance and
the amount of time at your disposal.

1.- With hands at sides or on hips, inhale and exhale
slowly and deeply, bringing the entire respiratory

apparatus into play.

2.- (To expand the chest and increase the air-capacity of the lungs)

Jerk the shoulders forward in several separate movements, inhaling deeper at each forward jerk. Exhale slowly, bringing the shoulders back to the original position.

Reverse the exercise, jerking the shoulders back-wards in similar manner while inhaling. Alternate the movements, forcing the shoulders first forward, them backwards.

3.- Stand erect, arms at sides. Inhale, raising the arms forward and upward until the palms touch above the head, at the same time raising on the toes as high as possible. Exhale, lowering the toes, bringing the hands downward in a wide circle until the palms touch the thighs.

4.- Stand erect, hands on hips. Inhale slowly, and deeply, raising the shoulders as high as possible, then, with a jerk, drop them as low as possible, let-ting the breath escape slowly.

5.- Stand erect, hands at shoulders. Inhale, raising elbows sideways; exhale, bringing elbows down so as to strike the sides vigorously.

6.- Inhale deeply, then exhale slowly, at the same time clapping the chest with the palms of the hands, covering the entire surface.

RHYTHMICAL BREATHING

It is a fact not generally known to us western people (our attention had to be called to it by the "Wise Men of the East."), that in normal rhythmical breathing exhalation and inhalation take place through one nostril at a time: for about one hour through the right nostril and then for a like period through the left nostril.

The breath entering through the right nostril
creates positive electro-magnetic currents, which pass
down the right side of the spine, while the breath
entering through the left nostril sends negative
electro-magnetic currents down along the left side
of the spine. These currents are transmitted by way
of the nerve centers or ganglia of the sympathetic
nervous system, which is situated alongside the spinal
column, to all parts of the body.

In the normal, rhythmical breath exhalation takes
about twice the time of inhalation. For instance, if
inhalation requires four seconds, exhalation, including a slight natural pause before the new inhalation,
requires eight seconds.

The balancing of the electro-magnetic energies
in the system depends to a large extent upon this
rhythimcal breathing, hence the importance of deep,
unobstructed, rhythmic exhalation and inhalation.

In order to establish the natural rhythm of the
breath when it has been impaired through catarrhal
affections, wrong habits of breathing, or other causes,
the following exercise, practiced not less than three
times a day (preferably in the morning upon arising,
at noon, and at night), will prove very beneficial
in promoting normal breathing and creating the right
balance between the positive and the negative electro-
magnetic energies in the organism.

THE ALTERNATIVE BREATH

Exhale thoroughly, then close the right nostril
and inhale through the left. After a slight pause
change the position of the fingers and expel the breath
slowly through the right nostril. Now inhale through
the right nostril and reversing the pressure upon the
nostrils exhale through the left.

Repeat this exercise from five to ten times,
always allowing twice as much time for exhalation as
for inhalation. That is, count three, or four, or six
for inhalation, and six, eight, ten, or twelve, respectively, for exhalation, according to your lung
capacity. Let your breaths be as deep and long as

possible, but avoid all strain.

This exercise should always be performed before an open window or, better yet, in the open air, and the body should not be constricted and hampered by tight or heavy clothing.

Alternate breathing may be practiced standing, sitting, or in the recumbent position. The spine should at all times be held straight and free, so that the flow of the electro-magnetic currents are not obstructed. If taken at night before going to sleep, the effect of this exercise will be to induce calm, restful sleep.

While practicing the "alternate breath," fix your attention and concentrate your power of will upon what you are trying to accomplish. As you inhale through the right nostril, will the magnetic currents to flow along the right side of the spine, and as you inhale through the left nostril, consciously direct to the left side the energies that have been built up.

There is more virtue in this exercise than one would expect, considering its simplicity. It has been in practice among the yogi's of the eastern countries since time immemorial.

> "For breath is the basis of the living organism's activity. Thus, such exercises may be beneficial or detrimental in their effect upon a body. Hence it is necessary than an understanding be had as to how, as to when, or in what manner such may be used." 2475-1

> "Then in the physical body there are those influences, then, through which each of these phases of an entity may or does become an active influence. There may be brought about an awareness of this by the exercising of the mind, through the manner of directing the breathing." 2475-1

Edgar Cayce was asked which of all the breathing exercises would be best for everyone to do. Of those that he gave the following ones are direct and reach the heart of the matter.

*"...the exercise that will expand the lungs,
raising the body at the same time to tiptoes
as much as possible, arms extended at right
angles from the body."* 304-3

*"Those that would be the activity to EVERY well
balanced body. Morning and evening exercises
with the full and deep inhalation, and quick
exhalation from the lungs; breathing in through
the nostrils and exhaling through the mouth
quickly."* 369-10

The wise men of India knew that with the breath
they absorbed, they took in not only the air elements,
but life itself. They have taught that this primary
force of all forces, from which all energy is derived,
ebbs and flows in rhythmical breath throughout all of
the created universe. Every living thing is alive by
virtue of and by partaking of this cosmic breath.

*"Breath itself--few ever consider the neces-
sity of breathing or the lack of same to keep
alive."* 3125-2

The more positive the demand, the greater the
supply. Therefore, while breathing deeply and rhyth-
mically in harmony with the universal breath, will to
open yourself more fully to the inflow of the life
force from the source of all life in the innermost
parts of your being.

This intimate connection of the individual soul
with the great reservoir of life must exist. Without
it life would be an impossibility.

A variation of the alternate nostril breathing
was given a number of times in the readings--and it is
also one of the standard yogi exercises that is very
energizing for the whole of the body.

*"In breathing, take into the right nostril,
strength! Exhale through thy mouth. Intake in
thy left nostril, exhaling through the right;
opening the centers of the body--if it is first*

*prepared to thine own understanding, thine own
concept of what ye would have if ye would have
a visitor, if ye would have a companion, if
ye would have thy bridegroom." 281-28*

*"Breathe in through the right nostril three
times, and exhale through the mouth. Breathe
in three times through the left nostril and
exhale through the right. Then, either with
the aid of a low music or the incanting of
that which carries self deeper--deeper--to the
seeing, feeling, experiencing of that image
in the creative forces of love, enter into the
Holy of Holies." 281-13*

Warning:

While the alternate breathing exercises are very
valuable for overcoming obstructions in the air passages, for establishing the habit of rhythmic breathing
and for refining and for accelerating the vibratory
activities on the physical, mental and spiritual planes
of being, they must be practiced with great caution.
These, and the other "Yogi" breathing exercises, are
very powerful means for developing abnormal psychic
conditions. They are therefore especially dangerous
to those who are already inclined to be physically and
mentally negative and sensitive. Such persons must
avoid all practices which tend to refine excessively
the physical body and to develop prematurely and,
abnormally the sensory organs or the spiritual centers
of the body. The most dangerous of all these methods
are a long extended fast, an unbalanced food diet and
sitting in the silence, as well as "Yogi breathing."
That is, sitting in darkness, in seclusion or in the
company of others with similar inclinations, keeping
the mind in a passive and receptive condition for the
extraneous impressions. These practices develop very
dangerous phases of abnormal and subjective psychism.

*"...these exercises are excellent, yet it is
necessary that special preparations be made*

--or that a perfect understanding be had by
the body as to what takes place when such
exercises are used.

"For BREATH is the basis of the living organism's activity. Thus, such exercises may be
beneficial or detrimental in their effect upon
a body."

"Hence it is necessary that an understanding be
had as to how, as to when, or in what manner such
may be used." 2475-1

"Q.- Just what preparation do you advice for
the body now?

"A.- This should be rather the choice of the
body, from its OWN development, than from what
ANY other individual, entity or source might
give.

"Purify the body, purify the mind; that the
principle, the choice of ideals as made by
the entity may be made manifest.

"Do whatever is required for this--whether the
washing of the body, the surrounding with this
or that influence, or that of whatever nature.

"As has been experienced, this opening of the
centers or the raising of the life force may
be brought about by certain characters of
breathing--for as indicated, the breath is
power in itself; and this power may be directed
to certain portions of the body. But for what
purpose? As yet it has been only to see what
will happen!

"Remember what curiosity did to the cat!

"Remember what curiosity did to Galileo, and
what it did to Watt--but they used it in quite
different direction in each case." 2745-1

CHAPTER NINETEEN

EXERCISE

PHILOSOPHY OF HEALTH

Next to overeating, lack of exercise as the natural way is one of the leading causes of weakness and ill health. This is true because nature in her wisdom has so planned the mechanics and physiology of animal life activity as essential in maintaining the normal conditions in the physical body.

In all preventative and curative work it is of the greatest importance that we study very carefully nature's laws and her methods, and so provide conditions as nearly as possible in harmony with them. In this we may derive much help by studying all of the wonderful correspondences between vegetable, animal and human life based on the unit of life, the primitive single cell.

In the plant kingdom we find that the activity, or exercise of the unit cell is provided for by wind, rain, and by changes in temperature and light. In the animal kingdom exercise is called forth by the search for food, by play and by the aggressive and defensive warfare. In the human kingdom exists the same necessity for activity, for human food, provision for shelter, in play, and in defense against nature's destructive forces and against animal and human enemies.

But man, loving leisure better than exertion and being a free moral agent, has followed the lines of least resistance. He enslaved the horse to draw his vehicles; invented railroad pullmans, automobiles, bicycles and all kinds of labor saving machinery in order to gain speed and to avoid the necessity for physical exertion. The unnatural conditions of civilized society have overburdened some with hard physical labor and condemned others to indoors and sedentary occupations compelling them to almost non-activity.

Systematic, corrective exercises are needed to counterbalance both extremes.

Most persons who have to work hard physically are under the impression that they need not take special exercise. This, however, is a mistake, and the reasons are obvious. It is necessary that the ill effects of such one sided activity be counteracted by exercise and movement that bring into active play all of the different parts of the body, especially those that are neglected during the working hours.

Hard gymnastics exercises such as weight lifting, boxing, wrestling and athletics feats which require great physical exertion are not conducive to normal development and longevity. On the contrary, the hard and severe physical labor, long continued gymnastics and athletic training overstimulate and overdevelop the muscular structures of the body at the expense of the vital organs and of the brain and nervous system. They cause the "muscle bound" condition which means congestion of the blood in the fleshy parts plus a deficiency in the vital organs, the brain and nervous systems of the body.

This tends to coarsen the body. The animal nature in time reveals itself in outward appearance by the coarsening of the features, by the disproportionate and distorted physique, and the stunted intellectual and esthetic development.

For these reasons the natural healing philosophy does not favor strenuous physical and physiological exercise, but advises lighter forms of physiological combined with psychological exercises.

PHYSICAL EXERCISE

Aside from breathing gymsnastics, general, or, in case of illness or deformity, special corrective and curative exercises should be taken every day.

Physical exercise has similar effects upon the system as hydropathic, massage, and osteopathic treatment. It stirs up those morbid accumulations in the tissues, stimulates the arterial and venous circulation, expands the lungs to their fullest capacity, thereby increasing the intake of oxygen, and most effectively promotes the elimination of the waste and morbid materials through skin, kidneys, bowels, and the respiratory tract.

Furthermore, well-adapted, systematic physical exercises tend to help correct dislocations of spinal vertebrae and other elements of the body structures. They relax and soften contracted and hardened muscles and ligaments, and "tone up" those tissues which are weakened and abnormally relaxed or too loose. Regular physical exercises means an increased blood supply, improved assimilation and better drainage for all of the vital organs of the body.

By means of systematic exercise, combined with deep breathing, the liberation and distribution of electro-magnetic energies in the system is also greatly promoted and attuned within the system itself.

Most persons who have to work hard physically are under the impression that they need not take special exercises. This, however, is a mistake. In nearly all kinds of physical labor only certain parts of the body are called into action and only certain sets of muscles exercised, while others remain totally inactive. This favors unequal development, which is injurious to the organism as a whole. It is most necessary that the ill effects of such one-sided activity be counteracted by exercises and movements that bring into active play all the different parts of the body, especially those that are neglected during the normal hours of work.

Systematic physical exercises are an absolute necessity for brain workers and those following such sedentary occupations. They not only need breathing gymnastics and corrective movements, each and every day, but should also take regular daily walks, under all kinds of weather conditions. Unless they do this faithfully, their circulation will become sluggish and their organs of elimination inactive. The cells and tissues of their bodies will gradually become clogged with morbid encumbrances, and this will inevitably lead to physical and mental deterioration. Cayce gave the following on exercise.

"It's well that each body, everybody, take exercise to counteract the daily routine activity so as to produce rest." 416-1

"Take more outdoor exercise, that--brings into play the muscular forces of the body. It isn't that the mental should be numbed, or should be cut off from their operations or activities --but make for a more evenly, a more perfectly balanced body-physical and mental...."341-31

"Then, be a well-rounded body. Take specific, definite exercises morning and evening. Make the body physically, as well as mentally tired, and those things which have been producing those conditions where sleep, inertia, poisons in the system from non-eliminations, will disappear--and so will the body respond to the diets." 341-31

Therefore:

"Best that every individual budget its time. Set so much time for study, so much time for relaxation, so much time for labor mentally, so much time for activity of the physical body, so much time for reading, so much time for social activities...each of these make for the creating of a better balance." 440-2

General rules:

1.- Weak persons and those suffering from malignant diseases, such as cancer, tuberculosis, heart trouble, asthma, or from displacements and ruptures, or who are liable to apoleptic seizures, etc., should not take any vigorous exercises except under the direction of a competent physician.

2.- At least twice a day all parts of the respiratory apparatus should be very thoroughly exercised. Deep breathing should accompany every corrective measure or

movement, whether it be a special breathing exercise
or not.

3.- Begin your exercises each day with light movements and change gradually to more vigorous ones, then
reverse the process, ending with light and relaxing
movements.

4.- When beginning to take systematic exercises, do
not make the separate movements too vigorous or continue them for too long. If any of them cause pain or
considerable strain, omit them until the body becomes
stronger and more flexible. The muscular soreness often
resulting from exercise at the beginning is, as a rule,
of little consequence and finally disappearing before
too long. The different movements should be practiced
in spite of it, because that is the only way to relieve
and overcome this condition.

5.- Stop when you begin to feel tired. Never overdo;
you should feel refreshed and relaxed after exercising,
not tired and shaky.

6.- Do not take vigorous exercise of any kind within
an hour and a half of eating, nor immediately before
meals. It is a good plan to rest and relax thoroughly
for about fifteen minutes before sitting at the table.

7.- Whenever practical, exercise out of doors. If
indoors, perform the movements near an open window or
where there is a current of fresh air flowing.

8.- Exercise undressed, if at all possible, or in a
regular gymnasium suit that gives free play to all
muscles. If dressed, loosen all tight clothing. Ladies
should wear their garments suspended from the shoulders by means of shoulder straps, or so-called reform
waists, the skirts being fastened to these.

9.- Always relax physically and mentally before taking
any of the physical exercises. This will create the
proper atmosphere for the coming activity.

10.- Apparatus is not necessary to produce results. However, dumbells may be used, but they should not be too heavy. One-pound dumbells are sufficiently heavy in most cases of exercising. The exercises described in the readings are intended for muscular control, flexibility and improvement of the circulation, and increased activity of the vital functions rather than for mere animal strength alone.

In the following paragraphs, we offer a minute selection of corrective movements as well as a few of those that were offered in the Cayce readings. The individual graduating from the more simple exercises to those requiring considerable agility and effort.

CORRECTIVE GYMNASTICS

1.- Raise the arms forward (at the same time beginning to inhale), upward above the head, and backward as far as possible, bending back the head and inhaling deeply. Now exhale slowly, at the same time lowering arms and head and bending the body downward until the fingers touch the toes. Keep the knees straight. Inhale again, raising arms upward and backward as before. Repeat from six to eight times.

2.- Inhale slowly and deeply, with arms at side. Now exhale, and at the same time bend to the left as far as possible, raising the right arm straight above the head and keeping the left arm close to the side of the body. Assume the original position with a quick movement at the same time inhaling. Exhale as before, bending to the right and raising the left arm. Repeat a number of times.
For making the chest flexible. Also excellent as stimulation for the organs of digestion.

3.- Chest stretcher: This exercise must be performed vigorously, the movements following one another in rapid succession.
Stand erect. Throw the arms backward so that the palms touch (striving to bring them higher with each

repetition), at the same time raising on the toes and inhaling. Without pausing, throw the arms forward and across the chest, the right arm uppermost, striking the back with both hands on opposite sides, at the same time exhaling and lowering the toes. Throw the arms back immediately, touching palms, rising on toes and inhaling as before, then bring them forward and across the chest again, left arm uppermost. Repeat from ten to twenty times.

An excellent massage and vibratory movement for the lungs and the chest.

4.- Stand erect, elbows to sides, hands closed on chest, thumbs inward. Thrust out the arms vigorously and quickly, first straight ahead, then to the sides, then straight up, then straight downward. Repeat each movement a number of times, then alternate them, each time bringing back arms and hands to the original position quickly and forcefully.

As a variation, raise the elbows sideways to shoulder-height with fists on shoulders, then strike vigorously as before, opening the palms and stretching the fingers with each thrust. Repeat anywhere, from ten to twenty times, or until tired.

For exercising the muscles of the chest and the upper arms.

5.- Stand erect, hands on hips. Keeping the legs straight, rotate the trunk upon the hips, bending first forward, then to the right, then backward, then to the left. Repeat a number of times, then rotate in the opposite direction.

Especially valuable for a sluggish liver.

6.- Lie flat on your back on a bed or, better still, a mat on the floor, hands under head. Without bending knees, raise the right leg as high as possible and lower it slowly. Repeat a number of times, then raise the other leg, then alternate. As the abdomen becomes stronger, raise both legs at once, keeping the knees straight. It is important that legs be lowered slowly.

For exercising the abdominal muscles and strength-

ening the pelvic organs. This exercise and the following one are especially valuable for remedying female
troubles.

7.- Lie flat on back, arms folded on chest. Place the
feet under a chair or bed to keep then in position.
Raise the body to a sitting posture, keeping knees,
back, and neck straight. Lower the body slowly to its
original position. Repeat from five to ten times,
according to your capabilities and strength.

SUPPLEMENTARY EXERCISES

8.- Stride-stand position (feet about one-half yard
apart). Raise the arms sideways until even with the
shoulders, then, without bending the back, rotate the
trunk upon the hips, first to the right, then to the left,
        As a variation of this exercise, rotate from the
waist only, keeping the hips motionless.
        An excellent massage for the intestinal organs.

9.- See-saw motion:
        Stride-stand position, arms raised sideways. Bend
to the right until the hand touches the floor, left arm
raised high. Resume original position. Repeat several
times, then bend to the left side, then alternate.

10- Chopping exercises:
        These are excellent for the abdominal walls.
        Stride-stand position. Clasp the hands above the
left shoulder. Swing the arms downward and between the
legs, bending well forward. Return to the original
position and repeat a number of times, then repeat with
hands on right shoulder, then alternate again.

11.- Cradle rock:
        Clasp hands over head, elbows straight. Bend the
trunk to the left and right side alternately and without
pausing a number of times.

12.- Stand erect, feet together. Jump to the stride-
stand position. at the same time raising arms sideways

to shoulders, jump back to original position and lower arms. Repeat from ten to twenty times.

13.- Lie flat on back, arms at side, legs straight. Raise both legs until they are at right angles with the body. From this position sway legs to the right and left side alternately.

14.- Lie flat on back, arms extended over head. Swing arms and legs upward simultaneously, touching the toes with the hands in mid-air, balancing the body on the hip bones and lower part of spine. Return to original position and repeat.

This is a difficult and strenuous exercise, and should not be attempted at first.

15.- Lie flat on stomach, hands over shoulders, palms downward, fingers turned inward, about six inches apart. This will give free play to the muscles of the chest. Raise the upper half of the body on the hands and arms as high as possible, keeping the body straight. Return to position and repeat until slightly fatigued.

16.- Same position as before. Raise the entire body on hands and toes, keeping arms and legs straight. Return to relaxed position and repeat the exercise.

As a variation, sway forward and backward while in the raised position.

17.- Lie flat on stomach, arms extended in front. Fling the arms upward and raise the upper part of the body as high as possible, keeping the legs straight. Return to position and repeat, but avoid excessive strain.

18.- Same position as before, put hands on hips or clasped in back. Raise upper part of body without assistance from hands or arms.

SPECIAL EXERCISES

19.- Lie flat on stomach, heels and toes together, hands stretched out in front. Fling head and arms upward, at the same time raising the legs, knees straight. Avoid any straining.

20.- Same position, hands clasped on back, feet together. Roll from side to side.

21.- Lie flat on back, seize a bar (bed rail or rung of a chair) just behind the head. Keeping the feet close together, raise the legs as high as possible, then swing them from side to side.. As a variation, swing legs in a circle flexing the knees.

22.- Same position. Raise and lower the legs up and down without letting them touch the floor, keeping the knees straight.

23.- Lie flat on back, fold the hands loosely across the stomach. Raise the lower and upper body without quite touching the floor.

24.- Stand erect, heels together, arms raised above the head. Bend forward and downward, endeavoring to place the palms on the floor in front of the body without flexing the knees. Return slowly to original position.

25.- Stand erect, hands on hips. Keeping the body motionless from the hips downward, sway the upper part of the body from side to side and forward and backward, and in a circle to right and left.

26.- Stand erect, raise the arms above the head. Rotate the trunk upon the hips with extended arms, bending as far as possible in each direction, but avoiding undue strain. These are very strenuous movements, they should not be carried to excess or performed for a long period of time.

    In practicing these exercises, it is always best to alternate them, that is, to select, say six or seven movements, as suited to individual conditions with a view to secure all-around general development and special practice for those parts and organs of the body that needs extra attention. The length of time at your disposal will also need to be considered.

Practice these exercises daily for a week. For the following week select six different exercises, then six more for the third week, and so on, supplementing the list given here with others, as suitable for your particular needs. Then start all over again in a similar manner.

This is better than doing the very same stunts each and every day. It promotes all-around development of the body and keeps the interest from dragging. Additional exercises are yet available in other Edgar Cayce materials and books as may be found in the local library or bookstore.

"We find that the exercise such as the setting-up exercise when the body first arises of a morning would be well, for this will bring strength to the lungs, vitality to the blood supply, and a new life, as it were, to the muscular forces of the body. Take then, at least five to ten minutes of exercises of the arms and limbs when the body first arises each mornings." 4462-1

"Mornings upon arising take for two minutes an exercise in this manner--where the body, standing with the feet flat on the floor, gently rises to the toes at the same time bringing the arms high above the head. Then bring these as far back as possible or practical, swinging both arms back. Breathe IN as the body rises and OUT as the body brings the hands to the front, slowly. Do this three or four times each morning...This is an excellent exercise for posture and for aiding in keeping this balance which will be set up by the general manipulations as combined with the osteopathic forces." 1773-1

"*Each morning before dressing, rise on tiptoe slowly and raise the arms easily at the same time (reaching) directly above the head, pointing straight up. At the same time, bend head back just as far as you can. When let down gentle from this, you see, we make for giving a better circulation, through the whole area from the abdomen through the diaphram, through the lungs, head and neck. Then let down, put the head forward, just as far as will come on the chest, then raise again at the top, bend the head to the right as far as it will go down. When rising again, bend the head to the left. Then standing erect, hands on hips, circle the head, roll around to the right two or three times, Then straighten self...will change all of those disturbances through the mouth, head and eyes, and the activity of the whole body will be improved.*" 470-37

"*Then in the morning before dressing, exercise the upper portion of the body; (by swinging) the arms up and down, straight up, straight down; then the turning motion as of swinging the arms around, for the movement...from the diaphram upward...from the ninth dorsal upward --these exercises will take away the heaviness, and the tendency to get tired easily.*"

2454-2

"*Be mindful that there is sufficient of the exercises that use the areas through the lumbar and sacral (regions); the bicycle riding, walking, horseback riding, rowing and the like.*"

1968-6

"*The exercises, particularly the setting up exercises, see? These be persistent with daily. Walking is good exercise, all outdoor activities such as tennis, croquet, riding, swimming. All of these are good but a few minutes morning and evening of the setting up exercises, at least three times each week the abdominal exercises.*" 1206-16

"Of mornings the body should rise early. First take the full setting up exercise of the body, upper and lower, circling the body from the hips up, bending from hips, stooping from hips, circling arms, head and neck." 137-1

"The best exercise for this body would be to stretch in the manner of a cat, or panther. Stretching the muscles but not straining them causes the tendons and muscles to be put into positions natural for the building of a strong and graceful body." 4003-1

"No better exercises may be taken than...the cat-stretching exercises, which includes, of course, being able--(put very coarsely) to do the split, be able to put the head on the feet, to put the feet behind the head, to make the head and neck exercises and all of those activities that may be said to be of the feline or cat exercise. To be sure, in the present period, present development, present conditions that exists, must be gone at gently; but be persistent morning and evening, working at it, still not letting it become rote, but purposeful." 681-2

Walking is the best exercise:

"Q.- What type of exercise is best for the body?
"A.- Walking is the best exercise. Bicycling --either stationary or in the open--is well. These are the better types of exercises. The open air activity is better." 2090-2

"Q.- How much walking should be done daily?
"A.- Whether if it is a mile or a step, do that which makes for a better 'feel' for the body; getting into the open!" 257-204

"Again let us give: Have a period for recreation, physically. Don't do this one day, or

*one day a week. If it is not capable of having
more than five minutes walk every day, do that!
That is better than an hour of strenuous exercise once a month, or even once in a week! There
is no better exercise than walking! Not fast,
but to be in the open, and to swing the body
in the movements—this is well for the body."*
257-217

*"Walking is good, especially in the open...
swimming is better than any. This is good, for
the activities of all the muscular forces are
brought into play in same." 920-11*

*"Those as would be indicated—walking is the
best exercise; of course, bending, or the
regular setting-up exercises are good."*
457-9

However:

*"These are as constant development for any
well being, well balanced body. Consistent
exercise with conditions as develop. Walking
exercise is well...yet these (exercises) must
ever be consistent with conditions as they
arise." 903-6*

Head and Neck exercises:

*"Yet with the general exercises—that is, the
circular motion of the head; backward; forward; to the sides—and with water, these
produce as it were a recharging of the battery
forces of the bodily functionings." 1554-4*

*"For those troublesome conditions with the
sympathetic system, if the body would take the
head and neck exercises, we will find it will
relieve those little tensions, which have been
indicated as part of the conditions in the
head, eyes, mouth and teeth...do not hurry
through with it, but take them regularly,
mornings—before dressing. 470-37*

"When we remove the pressures of the toxic forces we will improve the vision. Also the head and neck exercises will be most helpful. Take this regularly, not taking it sometimes and leaving off sometimes, but each morning and each evening take this exercise regularly for 6 months and we will see a great deal of difference; sitting erect, bend the head forward three times, to the back three times, to the right side three times, to the left side three times, and then circle the head each way three times. Don't hurry through with it but take the time to do it. We will get results."
3549-1

"Q.- How may my eyes be strengthened so as to eliminate reading glasses?

"A.- By the head and neck exercises in the open, as ye walk for twenty to thirty minutes each morning. Now do not undertake it one morning and then say 'It rained and I couldn't get out," or 'I've got to go somewhere else," --and think there aren't those despot conditions that rebel at not having their morning walk!" 2533-6

SPECIFIC EXERCISES

Hemorrhoids:

"But the best for the specific condition of hemorrhoids is the exercise, and if this is taken regularly these will disappear--of themselves! Twice each day, of morning and evening --and this doesn't mean with many clothes on rise on the toes, at the same time raising the arms; then bend forward, letting the hands go toward the floor. Do this three times of morning, and three times of evening. But don't do it two or three times and then quit, or don't do it three or four times a week and then quit, but do it regularly!" 2823-2

Better assimilations:

"The better change should come within from the better assimilation of that eaten which will be found to be more improved by the exercise of stretching arms above the head, or swinging on a pole would be well. This doesn't mean to run out and jump up on a pole every time you eat, but have regular periods. When you have the activities, do have these exercises, for they will stimulate the gastric flow and let that eaten have something to float in..." 2072-14

Abdomen exercise: the pelvic roll:

"The stretching of the abdomen as the exercise with feet against the wall; hands on the floor and raise and circle the body itself. This will keep the abdomen and the hips in correct position and keep body muscles through the hips and abdomen in such condition and positions as to make for much better activity in all the organs of the pelvis, the abdominal area." 1206-16

"...an exercise that will strengthen the whole condition of the spine, keep the abdominal muscles well as to general position of the body and keep the limbs in shape as to strengthen the muscles without being detrimental to any portion of the body...This will help the circulation, aid the digestion and improve the general conditions of the body." 308-13

Heavy legs:

"Standing flat upon the feet, gently rise upon the toes; do this for some six to eight to ten to fifteen times, gently; at the same time raising the arms gently with same during this, lower portion of the activities. This will

make for the proper circulation through those portions of the body." 412-10

"This is produced by impaired circulation through the lower extremities, produced by pressure existent in lower dorsal and lumbars. This may be aided materially by the right character of exercise and by keeping of eliminations as respecting the alimentary canal; exercise being such as takes the blood from the upper portion of the body, distributing same to lower portion, taking time to take specific exercises of stooping, bending and circular motions of mornings of the lower limbs, and then keeping up eliminations. This will correct condition." 417-2

To strengthen arches:

"The massage with the (specific) oils will be helpful. Also an exercise each day...would be well, of morning, before the shoes are put on --before the oil massage is given, of course (but do this daily); stand flat on the floor and spring on the toes, rising gently and springing." 3381-1

Feet:

"Rising upon the toes twice a day, morning and evening--upon arising and before retiring. Before putting on shoes and stockings of morning. Raise the arms, rocking back and forth on the heel and toe. Gradually, as the body raises up, raise the arms high also. Such an exercise is most beneficial." 1620-3

"It would be well if there would be this exercise night and morning; night before retiring--but after the massage as indicated, see; and of morning just before putting on the hose--after the massage has been given:

"Stand erect (without anything on the feet, of course). Then raise the arms, gently, slowly, over the head--directly over the head. Then gradually rise on the toes. Then as the body relaxes or lowers itself, lower the hands also--the hands extending in front of the body. Then rock back upon the heels, with the hands extended sufficiently to strain or to exercise the bursa of the heel, or those portions of the heel AND the arch, you see, to aid in strengthening. Doing this, together WITH the massage of the properties indicated through heel and arch, and especially over the frontal portions of the foot, we will bring better conditions for same." 1771-3

Conclusion:

"Common or ordinary understanding should give one the correct idea as to how the application of exercise deals with the body; if a little thought is given to this: That the body is built up by the radiation of vibratory forces from each and every unit of the body functioning in its proper manner.
"Then to overexercise any portion not in direct need of same, to the detriment of another, is to hinder rather than to assist through exercise. Exercise is wonderful and necessary, and little or few take as much as is needed, in a systematic manner. Use common sense, use discretion." 283-1

Therefore:

"The best way to acquire the correct amount of pep is to take the exercise." 200-38

CHAPTER TWENTY

AIR AND LIGHT BATHS

Even among the adherents of natural healing there are those who think that air and light baths should be taken out of doors in warm weather only, and in winter months only in well-heated rooms.

This is a mistake. The effect of the air bath upon the organism is subject to the same law of action and reaction which governs the effects of water applications.

If the temperature of air and water is the same or nearly the same as that of the body, no reaction takes place, the conditions within the system remain the same. But if the temperature of air or water is considerably lower than the body temperature there will be a reaction.

In order to "react" against the chilling effect of cold air or water, the nerve centers which control the circulation send the blood to the surface in large quantities, "flushing" the skin with warm, red arterial blood. The flow of the blood stream is greatly accelerated, and the elimination of morbid matter on the surface of the body is correspondingly increased.

POOR SKIN ACTION

Man is naturally an air animal. He breathes with the pores of the skin as well as with the lungs. However, the custom of hiding under dense and heavy clothing, thus excluding it from those life-giving influences of air and light, together with the habit of warm bathing, has weakened and enervated the skin of the average individual until it has lost all its tonicity and is no longer capable of fulfilling its natural functions.

The compact, almost air-tight layers of underwear and outer clothing made of cotton, wool, silk, and leather, prevent the ventilation of the skin and the escape of morbid excretions of the body. The skin is an organ of absorption as well as of excretion; consequently the systemic poisons which are eliminated from the organism, if not removed by proper ventilation and bathing, are reabsorbed into the system just like the poisonous exhalations from the lungs are reinhaled and reabsorbed by people congregating in closed rooms or sleeping in unventilated bedrooms.

Who would think of keeping plants or animals continuously covered up, away from the air and light? We know that they would wither and waste away, and die before any length of time passed.

Nevertheless, civilized human beings have for ages hidden their bodies most carefully from sun and air, which are so necessary for their well-being. Is it any wonder that the human body has become withered, enervated, and atrophied, that it has lost the power to perform freely and efficiently its functions of elimination and absorbtion? Undoubtedly, this has to do with the prevalence of all kinds of diseases.

On awakening in the morning and several times during the day, if circumstances permit, expose your nude body to the invigorating influences of the open air and sunlight.

Not only should we sleep with our bedroom window open year-round, but if at all possible, air baths should be taken out of doors. Every house should have facilities for air and sun baths, that is, an enclosed area where the nude body can be exposed to the open air and the sunlight.

If the air bath out of doors is impractical, it may be taken in front of an open window. But indoor air, even in a well ventilated room, is more or less stagnant and vitiated, and at best only a poor substitute for the open air of the outdoors.

It is the breezy, moving outdoor air permeated with sunlight and rich in oxygen and ozone that generates the electric and magnetic currents which are so stimulating and vitalizing to everything that draws the breath of life.

This important fact is now being realized more

and more, and air-bath facilities will in the very near future be considered as indispensable in modern up-to-date homes as is the bathroom today.

It is suggested, in the beginning, to expose the nude body to cool air only for short periods of time until the skin becomes inured to it.

Likewise, unless you are well used to the sun, take air baths of short duration, that is, from ten to twenty minutes, until your skin and nervous system have become accustomed to the influence of heat and strong light. Prolonged exposure to the glaring rays of the sun might produce severe burning of the surface of the skin, aside from a possible harmful effect to the nervous system.

> *"Q.- What quantity of sunbathing should the body take to replace ultraviolet (lamp)? Or should the body take both?*
> *"A.- No. We would take the sun-bath, but take that which adds to the body. Do not tan the body too much! That which gives the full activity to the capillaries, or to the exterior portions of the system is fine."* 275-20

> *"Keep (the child) in the open often, but never with the sun shining directly on the face or eyes. These should ever be shaded....It is the absorption of the ultra-violet which gives strength and vitality to the nerves and muscular forces, which come from the effect of the rays of the sun on or from the activities of the body. It is not well that there be too much tan from the sun on the body. This forms on the body to protect the body from same. Thus not too much tan, but sufficient for the healthy activity of the body."* 3172-2

Warning:

> *"Q.- What is the cause of the injury to the eyes?*
> *"A.- Too strong a light when very young--in sunlight."* 5126-1

"Take as much outdoor exercise as is possible in sunshine. Should the sunshine seem to produce headaches and strain on eyes, these conditions will be found to be remedied by wearing dark glasses or shading the eyes. The vitality as caused from the sun will be effective toward vitalization of the body." 81-2

The novice should protect the head and eyes against the fierce rays of sunlight. This is best accomplished by means of a wide-brimmed straw hat of light weight. In cases where dizziness results from the effect of the heat upon the brain, a wet cloth may be swathed around the head or placed inside the straw hat.

It will be found very pleasurable and also very invigorating to take a cold shower or spray, off and on during the sunbath, and allow the air to dry the body. This will also increase its electro-magnetic effects upon the system.

FRICTION BATH

While taking the air bath, the skin may be rubbed or brushed with a rough towel or a flesh brush in order to remove the excretions and the atrophied cuticle. The friction bath should always be followed by a spray or a cold-water rub.

At the time of the air bath, practice breathing exercises and the curative gymnastics appropriate to your condition.

If the air bath is taken at night, before retiring, the less active breathing exercises may be taken with good results, but all vigorous stimulating movements should be avoided.

As the plant prospers under the life-giving influence of light and water, so the cuticle of the human skin becomes alive under the natural stimulation of water, air, and sunlight. From the foregoing paragraphs it will be seen why the air and light bath is regarded as one of the most important natural methods of treatment in all of nature's methods of treatment and curative powers.

"Q.- What changes in civilization cause us to be unlikely to get enough sunshine vitamin D as nature originally intended?
"A.- The tendency to have less sunshine activity, or less activity in the sunshine, and the taking of more foods that are not close to nature.
"Q.- Why do the members of my family absolutely need a constant and plentiful supply of sunshine vitamin D, especially right now?
"A.- The lack of sunshine at the present season, the necessity for the structural portions or frame portions of the body. These add, or this vitamin adds, to that necessary element in the structural building of the body, that is lacking when sunshine is not as plentiful as to the present time.
"Q.- How does sunshine vitamin D help to insure better teeth, stronger bones, and the general well-being of my family?
"A.- Adding those necessary elements for the building, especially, of those structural portions of the body." 658-11

However:

"Let there not be too much activity in the middle of the day, or too much (of) the sunshine. The early mornings and the late afternoons are the more preferable times. For the sun during the period between eleven or eleven-thirty and two o'clock carries too great a quantity of the actinic rays that make for destructive forces to the superficial circulation..." 934-2

That is, during the hot season of the year and in tropical countries the best time for taking air and sun baths is the early morning and the late afternoon.

Persons suffering from insomnia or nervousness in any form are in nearly every case greatly benefited by a short air bath taken just before retiring.

Physical labor and exercise will also help cure that known as sleeplessness or insomnia.

> *"Q.- What is the best way for me to get to sleep?*
> *"A.- Labor sufficiently--at work of a physical nature--to tire the body; not mentally, but physically." 2067-1*

> *"Q.- Why can't I sleep at night?*
> *"A.- This is from nervousness and over-anxiety. Of course keep away from any drugs if possible, though a sedative at times may be necessary. Drink a glass of warm milk with a teaspoonful of honey stirred in it." 2514-7*

And here follows one of the most, if not the most important aspect of healing given in the Edgar Cayce readings and which has not been even considered by any, let alone known.

> *"Sleep is a sense (like the five senses), as we have given heretofore, and it is that which is needed for the physical body to recuperate, or to draw strength from the mental and spiritual powers or forces that are held as the ideals of the body.*
> *"Don't think that the body is a haphazard machine, or that the things which happen to individuals are chance! It is all a law! Then, what happens to a body in sleep? That is dependent upon what it has thought, what it has set as its ideal!*
> *"For when one considers, one may find these as facts: there are individuals who in their sleep gain strength, power, might because of their thoughts, their manner of living. There are others who find that when any harm, any illness, any dejection comes to them, it is following sleep! It is again a matter of following a law!*
> *"What happens to this particular body? That*

is dependent upon the manner it has applied itself during those periods of its waking state. Take time to sleep! It is the exercising of a faculty, a condition, that is meant to be a part of the experience of each soul. It is as but the shadow of life, or lives or experiences in the earth, just as each day of an experience is part--a part of the whole that is being builded by an entity, a soul. And each night is as but a period of putting away, a storing up, into the superconscious or the unconsciousness of the soul itself."
                                                    2067-1

"Concentration upon relaxation is the greater or better manner of any body to relax. That is, see the body relaxing, consciously! Not by concentrating so as to draw in the (spiritual) influences, but in such a way as to let all of the tension, all of the strain, flow out of self--and find the body giving, giving away."
                                                    404-5

Therefore:

"Then in the material self, make it a habit, make it a hobby, to at least each day speak kindly to someone less fortunate than self. Not that there should be so much the contribution to organized charity, but have those charities of self you never speak of, by speaking kindly to someone each day. This will let the body rest at night when it hasn't been able to, with its mental and material worries.
                                                    5177-2

"Q.- Why can't I get a decent night's sleep and what should I do about it?
"A.- Take the treatments of hydrotherapy and massage at least, as given, once or twice a week, but extend them over a long period... after those indicated periods of recreation or rest or change. Then when the body returns from such periods have a few more, every week or so have at least one or two of these, for

*varied periods, and we will find much bettered
conditions. But don't forget, as the Boy Scout
or Girl Scout oath would be: Do a good deed
every day. This is just being kind, just being
patient, showing long-suffering, gentleness!
And we will find much help for this body!"*
5177-1

And:

*"Q.- Is it best to have windows open or closed
while sleeping at night?
A.- Top and bottom of windows should be
opened." 4008-1*

OUTDOOR EXERCISE

*"Those that have most to do with the outside,
no matter what season or portion of the year.
As they change (the seasons), those that have
most to do with the outside; for, as just
given, in the elements the interesting factors
are earth and fire--while air and water are
rather matters of course to the entity! yet in
its studies, and in its developments, its
factors will be brought out. Hence on the earth
and in the air bring for a balance that will
keep those same elements, or forces, in the
proper activity and balance through the mental,
spiritual, and physical forces of the body.
"Q.- Any special sports?
"A.- All those that have to do with the out-of-
doors, whether it be in the spring or the summer
or the rowing, or in the fall the first of the
golfing--these those of the heavier, or sking,
or sliding, or sledding, or the like." 488-6*

*"Hence we find again that sports, and the
outdoor life and activities, are a part of
the present urges; yet the appreciation of the
influence of such for body-development, body-
building, as well as for supplying entertain-
ments and activities for individuals and
groups alike." 1074-2*

*"One with the inclination for the activities
of the body to produce too great avoirdupois.
Hence precautions become necessary as to the
activity of the glands, and a greater part of
the entity's diet should be citrus fruits.*
*"Also there should be a greater activity (that
arises from inclinations once set in motion)
for every form of outdoor sports; especially
walking, golfing, archery, riding, boating,
tennis--and all outdoor sports that tend to
keep not only beauty of figure bodily but to
give--as will be seen--the expressing of self
in those activities that answer to emotions,
intuitively, in the entity." 1346-1*

*"Well to keep the general activity, the exer-
cise. And do have some of that each day in the
open, when practical. There is more value in
exercising in the sun than many a dose, or
even at times meditation." 272-12*

THE IMPORTANCE OF SKIN AS
AN ORGAN OF ELIMINATION

Of late physiologists have claimed that the skin
is not of any great importance as an organ of elimination. Common experience and the diagnosis from the
eye teach us differently. The black rim seen more or
less distinctly in the outer rim of the iris in the
eyes of the majority of people, has been called the
"scurf rim," because it was found that this dark rim
appeared in the iris after the suppression of scurvy
and other forms of skin eruptions: and was after the
external or internal use of lotions, ointments and
medicines containing mercury, zinc, iodine, arsenic,
or other poisons which suppressed or destroyed the
life and activity of the skin.

Therefore, when we see in the iris of a person
a heavy scurf-rim, we can tell the person at that very
moment: "Your cuticle is in a sluggish and atrophied
condition, the surface circulation and eliminations
through the skin are not good, and as a result of this

there is a strong tendency to auto-intoxication, you take cold easily, and suffer from chronic catarrhal conditions. Therefore, a heavy scurf-rim frequently indicates what is called a "scrofulous condition."

This certainly shows the great importance of the skin as an organ of elimination, and the necessity of keeping it in the best possible condition. It explains why an atrophied skin has such a great deal to do with the causation of disease, and why in the treatment of both acute and chronic ailments air and cold water produce such wonderful results.

"Q.- What should be done to clear the skin?
"A.- The combination of things as we have indicated. First the Atomidine will tend to make for the coordinating of the channels of elimination. The skin condition is rather from the improper coordinating of the activities through the peristaltic movement, or absorption in the torso of the body. Thus it produces a condition wherein the irritations are being produced from the poisons being eliminated through the perspiratory system rather than through alimentary canal." 2579-1

Therefore, the skin as an organ of elimination suffers when the bowels are functioning improperly. The concept in the readings states that poor elimination by the skin is caused when eliminations through the enteric tract are inadequate.

"Q.- What treatment to stimulate eliminations?
"A.- These are best stimulated by the diet and exercise. As has been in those given, these in the diet should be that as is a mild laxative, rather than cathartics, see? and when there is the tendency of this condition to become sluggish, those of oils--preferably much more of olive than just plain mineral oil. For olive oil--properly taken--is a food for the intestinal tract. This would be well to be considered by many: That, that may be assimilated by the system--of olive oil--pure--is

*food value for the system itself, and tends
to stimulate peristaltic movements, see? Taken
then, in very small quantities--but rather
often, and when found to disagree--or a tendency, from the foods or the character of
drinks taken--discontinue: for nothing is more
severe than rancid, or oil that has become
over acted on by the hydrochlorides in the
system. Only that as will assimilate. So olive
oil or mineral oil--in moderation: but diet
and exercise the best."* 5603-5

*"Q.- What is the cause of my skin eruptions
that I have so frequently, and kindly give me
a cure for same?
"A.- These are part of the circulatory disturbance, and as the eliminations are set up and
as there are coordinations between the forces
in the body itself that makes for a coordinant
reaction in all portions of the eliminations,
we will find these disturbances being eliminated."* 603-3

*"Q.- What is still causing my face and neck
to break out in pimples and what can be done
to cure them completely?
"A.- These will disappear if the corrections
are made properly and the eliminations are
kept well."* 3081-3

*"Q.- How may I best clear up my complexion?
"A.- By increasing or stimulating the general
circulation for coordination in the eliminations."* 1101-4

*"First, in the blood supply we find indications
of the inclination toward poor eliminations
through the alimentary canal; and this is
inclined to produce toxic forces that cause
a poor coordination between the superficial
and the deeper circulation.
"Hence those disturbances as a rash, or black-*

*heads, or pimples, or large pores—all of these
are at times indicated."* 2154-2

*"Q.- What can be done locally for impurities
on my face?
"A.- ...keep the eliminations open."* 452-2

*"Q.- What can be done to clear up the skin?
"A.- Make for the better eliminations."*
2071-2
480-22

However:

*"Q.- I am a lover of beauty, and without
vanity—would like to make myself more beautiful. How can I.?
"A.- Through those same channels that the
entity gained this understanding that beauty
comes from within, rather than as an external
condition—for the external fades, but that
beauty of life, of individuality shining
through that personality of self, gives the
beauty that fades not—and as the warning was
given respecting the understanding of self; and
that to be accomplished through the efforts
of self, these must radiate then from within.
"As to the physical appearance, and the outward
show of face and figure, necessary that these
be modeled after that of the self's ideal, that
these may manifest that the body would radiate
through its inner being. Accomplish this
through that of self's own application to
become that the body would make of self....
Seek that satisfaction of self being at an
at-oneness with that beauty of the creative
energies for the benefit of others, and not
of self."* 2071-2

Therefore:

*"As for scars, rather let the scars be removed
from the mental and spiritual self. To undertake such through those activities of anyone*

altering these, we will have worse scars. Let
the scars be removed from the own mental, the
OWN MENTAL AND SPIRITUAL SELF. Turn to those
things of making application of the fruits of
the spirit of truth: love, patience, gentle-
ness, kindness, long-suffering, brotherly
love, putting away those little tendencies
for being "catty" at times or being selfish
or expressing jealousy and such. Let that mind
be in thee as was in Him, who is the way and
the truth and the light, and He will make the
light of love so shine through thy countenance
that few, if any, will ever see the scars made
by self-indulgence in other experiences."
"Q.- What can be done to correct excessive oil-
iness which has resulted in acne and scarring?
"A.- Just read what we have been giving."

                                        5092-1

Regular outdoor (in the open air) work, sufficient
to produce good perspiration, where one is in close
touch with Mother Nature, is the best of all exercise
for human beings. The work itself should be constructive
to the extent that it provides some of the necessities
of human life and calls forth the best instincts of
human nature. There is none better than the tilling
of the soil for the production of vegetables, fruits,
herbs and flowers.

"All that is for the sustenance of life IS
produced from the soil. Then there must be a
return to the soil. Every man must be in that
position that he at leasts creates, by his
activities, that which will sustain the body."

                                        3976-19

Elimination through perspiration produced by the
vigorous outdoor work, bareheaded and barefooted, is by
all means the best of all. Such natural activity is
best done before eating.

Numerous experiments have demonstrated that
perspiration resulting from actual work or play is
far more effective in the elimination of morbid matter
from the human body than perspiration induced by steam

baths, hot air, or other artificial contrivances. It
is also true that actual outdoor exercise in the shape
of constructive work or play produces much better
results than exercise taken with special apparatus in
heated buildings.

Next to tilling the soil, outdoor play is one
of the best forms of exercise as brought out in the
readings, such outdoor games bring into activity the
whole muscular system and provides the best possible
exercise for the lungs, the heart and the vital organs,
while at the same time it calls forth intense brain
activity, coordination and concentration of mind by
such competition and rivalry.

*"The body should be in the open as much as
possible. Not too strenuous exercise, but
sufficient that the whole organism of the body
is affected by the exercise; that is, such
exercise--whether as of specific in mornings
and evenings, or outdoors--as golf, or riding,
or rowing, or swimming, or such--that require
the use of all the muscular forces of the
system. These should be taken by the body.
Not too strenuous, but sufficient to keep
these active with those conditions as will be
changed in the vibratory forces of the body.
"Following such, to be sure--that is, such
treatments--or such exercise--the body should
be rubbed down thoroughly, and a gentle massage
--either osteopathically or neuropathically,
or Swedish massage--given all over the body,
that the distribution of the changes in the
vibratory forces of the body, as well as the
circulatory system, should be stimulated
throughout. We will find this will aid much
that condition as has been seen in feet, as
well as that which has been in head and neck,
and throat. These will be aided by these
changes, for these are effects--not causes--
in the system."* 5602-1

Next to outdoor sport, the best natural form of

exercise is walking. To attain the best results walks
should be taken not alone but in company with some
congenial companion. Select some objective point and
make the walk vigorous and rapid, the arms swinging
free from the shoulders, the breathing deep and vigorous, the carriage of the body erect. Now and then
take a "chest lift." This is done while walking. Hold
the entire body erect, draw in a breath; after a few
seconds, without exhaling, draw in another and after
a further interval of a few seconds, still another.
After the third inhalation vigorously expel all the
air. The object of this is to inflate the chest to
its fullest capacity.

Four or five miles are not too much for a good
vigorous walk, although one or two miles a day may be
all the average city dweller can afford. To get the
best results from any form of exercise the clothing
should be removed immediately afterward and a cold rub
or cold sponge bath taken, followed by a brisk rub
with a dry towel. This in turn should be followed by
a few minutes rest or thorough relaxation in order
to allow the system to resume its normal functions.

Since a large proportion of people who live in
cities find it absolutely impossible in their regular
life to take natural exercise in the shape of work,
play or walking, they must have some substitute in the
way of indoor exercise. Many people believe that the
chief object of exercise is to develop large muscles
and unusual strength, and for that purpose all kinds
of special apparatus, weights and many other various
contrivances have been devised and sold at fancy fees.

Such apparatus is entirely unnecessary for good
physical development and for maintaining good normal
health. The leading authorities on physical culture
agree that best results may be obtained by the simple
exercises, resisting tensing and relaxing, without the
use of weights or special apparatus.

Exercising in order to produce best results must
be regular. Set aside a certain time each day for this
purpose and adhere to it. The body becomes accustomed
to duties of this kind, performed at regular times
each day. The entire reserve forces of the organism

is brought into play at these times and great benefit
is derived not only from the physical effects but also
from the concentration of mind and will on the work
in hand, and this will gradually extend to all other
forms of physical and mental occupations.

*"Then, in making helpful suggestions for
activities of the body--we find those activities are well that keep a better balance in
the superficial and the deeper circulation,
keeping much of those poisons from the system;
that is, poisons from the energies of the body.
Wherever, whenever there are those activities
mentally OR physically, there must necessarily
be the used energies, as in the discharge of
the dead cells of blood supply, whether white
or red blood or leucocyte. These must be
eliminated. With the catabolism disturbed,
these become as ash, or poisons: not to the
point--as yet--of a toxic condition, or a
poisoning of that nature, but those tendencies.
"Hence hydrotherapy, with the light sweats,
good rubdowns, and the occasional cleansing
of the colon, would be manners to bring
coordination." 2091-3*

CHAPTER TWENTY-ONE

MANIPULATIVE TREATMENTS

MASSAGE

Massage has very much the same effects upon the system as the cold water treatment. It accelerates the circulation, draws the blood to the surface, relaxes and opens the pores of the skin, promotes the elimination of morbid matter, and increases and stimulates the electro-magnetic energies in the body.

We have learned that one of the primary causes of chronic disease is the accumulation of waste matter and systematic poisoning of the tissues of the body. These morbid encumbrances clog the capillaries, thus obstructing the circulation and interfering with or preventing the normal activity of the organs of elimination, especially the skin.

The in depth massage, the squeezing, kneading, rolling, and stroking, actually squeezes the stagnant blood and the morbid accumulations out of the tissues into the venous circulation, speeds the venous blood, charged with waste matter products and poisons, on its way to the lungs, and enables the arterial blood with its freight of oxygen and nourishing elements to flow more freely into the less obstructed tissues as well as the organs.

Through manipulation of the fleshy tissues, the blood is drawn to the surface of the body, and in that way the elimination of the morbid matter through the relaxed and opened pores of the skin is then greatly facilitated.

"The blood supply being that in the system which performs, through its various channels, more than one function--for the supply retains and attains, from the assimilation of foods in system, for the replenishing of the body,

*as well as often acting as a carrier for
elimination of used energies to their various
portions or conditions in system where such
eliminations may take place; performing also
that function of being able to create that
which acts as the coagulating forces for the
body in any condition as may be occurrent, or
concurrent in the system. Hence, this often
may be classified as that criterion through
which most any condition existent in the system
may be found." 108-2*

*"...there is no condition existent in a body
that the reflection of same may not be traced
in the blood supply, for not only does the
blood stream carry the rebuilding forces to
the body; it also takes the used forces and
eliminates same through their proper channels
in the various portions of the system. Hence
we find red blood, white blood and lymph and
carried in the veins. These are only separated
by the very small portions that act as builders,
strainers, destroyers or resuscitating portions of the system...Hence there is ever seen
in the blood stream the reflection or evidences
of that condition being carried on in the
physical body. The day may yet arrive when one
may take a drop of blood and diagnose the
condition of any physical body." 283-2*

Therefore:

*"...the circulation, or the blood...is the
main attribute to the physical body, or that
which keeps life in the whole system, or body,
in itself." 4614-1*

And:

*"As is understood by the body, there is within
each organ that ability to take from the system
that necessary for the rebuilding of itself,*

the continuous reproduction of itself...Here
we find hindrances in the circulation. True,
impulse for physical consciousness reacts from
nerve centers of the brain, but the supply of
nourishment--as well as the ability of portions
of the organs to receive that assimilated--
comes from BLOOD supply, that is controlled
by the ganglia along the nervous system--either
the cerebro-spinal or the sympathetic."

1158-31

"...for while the blood is the life-giving
factor from that as is assimilated by the body,
it must go through that form or process within
the body itself for the use of same in building,
in replenishing, or in resuscitating life-
giving forces." 2884-1

The human body as an electrical machine requires
a storage battery, wires and machinery for movement.
The primary storage battery is in the form of thousands
of ganglionic cells whose sole duty is to store away
the electrical energies of the body; the complicated
system of wires is in the form of nerves, whose sole
duty is to transmit the electrical fluid from the ganglionic cells to the muscles or other parts; a set of
machinery in the form of muscles, organs, and bones.
The nerve-system, the main parts thus roughly
examined, effects the motions and sensations of the
body, and is that system that supplies energies to
the various parts of the body, the organs and centers
of mobility. The association of the nervous system to
that of the circulatory system is as immense as is the
significance of their relationship to each other for
maintaining the equilibrium. The massage, of course,
affects both of these systems in a most dramatic and
effective manner.

"The massage is very well, but we would do
this the more often, see? As long as there is
an opportunity of it producing the effect to
all areas of the better activity to the organs
of the body. The 'why' of the massage should

be considered: Inactivity causes many of these
portions along the spine from which impulses
are received to the various organs to be lax,
or taut, or to allow some to receive greater
impulse than others. The massage aids the
ganglia to receive impulse from nerve forces
as it aids circulation through the various
portions of the organism." 2456-4

"...the 'batteries' of the nervous system are
running down; that is, the activities of the
heart, the lungs, the liver, the kidneys may
be called the batteries of the body. With
changes in the chemical forces of the system,
these may become so reduced in their activity
as to cause stress to be put upon one or the
other, thus gradually building a disturbance
functionally. With the distress or disturbance
(thus produced), one or the other (organ)
gradually becomes organically disordered."
                                        4007-1
"Then we find that the nervous system must be
taken into consideration, as to how the very
active force of the blood supply itself is
taken, for with each muscular force of the
body, and with practically all change in the
blood supply, whether of the active force as
returns the blood to the heart or takes it
from the heart, must receive an impulse from
same to function in a normal manner. Then,
when we have hindrances--as is designated or
seen here with this body, where nerves fail
to receive proper incentives, the reaction from
those organs or those portions of the system
supplied by that nerve energy suffers in its
cycle of functioning." 108-2

Therefore:

"...hydrotherapy and massage are preventative
as well as curatives measures. For the cleansing
of the system allows the body-forces themselves

> *to function normally, and thus eliminate poi-*
> *sons, congestions and conditions that would*
> *become acute throughout the body." 257-254*

Very important are the electro-magnetic effects
of good massage upon the system. The positive magnetism
of the operator will stir up and intensify the latent
energies in the body of the patient, very much like
a piece of iron or steel is magnetized by rubbing it
with a horseshoe magnet. The more normal and positive
morally and mentally, as well as physically, the operator, the more marked will be the good effects of the
treatment upon the weak and negative patient.

> *"As we find here, the relaxings of the body by*
> *or through suggestions made as to almost hypno-*
> *tize the body, will help. This should be done*
> *by the power of suggestion, at the same time*
> *that applications would be made for magnetic*
> *healing. This may be done by the very close*
> *associates of the body.*
> *"Place the right hand (of the one making appli-*
> *cation) on the back, opposite the pit of the*
> *cardiac portion of the stomach and the left hand*
> *over the cardiac portion of the stomach. Hold*
> *for three or four minutes. This should be direc-*
> *tly on the body, not through the clothing. At*
> *the same time, there should be those suggestions*
> *for the increasing of the flow of blood, the*
> *increasing of the flow of nerve forces, as to*
> *relieve these tensions that have been produced.*
> *"These forms or manners will be much preferable*
> *to attempting to use counter-irritants with any*
> *form of plaster, mustard plaster, or...where...*
> *other characters of counter-irritants are used.*
> *It will be well that this be done at least once*
> *each day for at least fifteen or eighteen days."*
> *   3619-1*

The beneficial effects of magnetic treatment is
not so much due to the actual transmission of vital
force from operator to patient as to the arousing and
stimulating of the latent, inactive electro-magnetic

energies of the latter, the "polarizing" of its own magnetic forces.

Neither does the horseshoe magnet impart its own magnetism to the piece of iron which is rubbed with it, but the electro-magnetic energies in the magnet arouses to vibratory activity the latent electro-magnetic energies in the iron. This is proved by the fact that both magnet and iron will remain magnetic as long as they are used for magnetizing other substances, but that both will lose their magnetic qualities through dis-use or dis-ease.

It is true that manipulative work, like everything else, can be overdone and produce harmful effects upon the operator. But within reasonable limits, massage and magnetic treatments will not deplete the person giving them, providing his or her system is kept in good condition. His own vibrations must be harmonious on all planes of being, the physical, mental, moral, and spiritual. The individual must be inspired and actuated by the faith that he can heal by the positive attitude of will to heal, and by being in sympathy with the one he is trying to benefit.

Such an operator makes himself the instrument or channel for the transmission of life force, which is "healing" force, from the source of all life. "As he gives, so he receives"; for this is the basic law of the universe, the Law of Compensation. If he gives the treatments in the right spirit, he will gain vital force instead of losing it. He will actually feel his own force intensified, and after the treatment he will experience a feeling of buoyancy and of elation which nothing else can impart to him.

> *"For no element outside of the body produces healing, but that the attunement to the coordinating and cooperative forces of life-force as it meets the various influences that have been brought about by some error or some misapplication, the awareness of the God-Force, the Life-Force working in and through the system." 1173-8*

Therefore:

*"...all building and replenishing for a
physical body is from within, and must be
constructed by the mind of the entity; for
Mind is the Builder; for each cell in the
atomic force of the body is as a world of its
own, and each one--each cell--being in perfect
may build to that necessary to reconstruct
the forces of the body in all its needs..."*
93-1

The above applies to the patient as well as to
the healer or manipulator. Good massage will produce
electro-magnetic effects through the operator is not
aware of it and does not understand the underlying laws;
but his work will gain in power and effectiveness and
in direct proportion to the conscious efforts he makes
to benefit his patients by the influence of those inner
invisible forces.

The electro-magnetic energies of the organism can
be controlled by the will and either concentration to
or sent away from any part of the body, just as the
circulation of the blood can be controlled. I saw the
latter done by a hypnotist who made the blood flow into
and out of the arms and hands of one of his subjects
simply by the power of will alone.

While this was accomplished by means of that
destructive process, it has taught me a most valuable
lesson regarding the power of will to control physical
conditions or activities of others.

*"Here we have an emotional body well versed
in the study of meditation, the study of
transmission of thought, with the ability to
control others.*
*"Don't control others. Suppose thy God control-
led thee without thy will? What would you
become, or what would you have been?*
*"But you were made in the image of the Creator,
to be a companion with Him--not over someone
else, but a companion with thy brother and not
over thy brother. Hence do not act that way,*

*because ye have the greater ability or greater
knowledge of control of others."* 3428-1

It is obvious that magnetic treatment or massage
will not remove pain permanently if the latter is due
to irritation caused by a luxated bone, or by some
foreign body, or by local accumulation of morbid matter
and poisons in any part of any organ. In all such cases
the local cause of that irritation must be removed,
before any of the pain can subside or disappear altogether. Pain is just an effect of something wrong in
the functioning of the organism.

*"Q.- How can arthritis of left hip, lower
vertebra and hands be lessened?*
*"A.- By the application of heating oils; as
the Camphorated Oil, and a combination of Olive
Oil and Tincture of Myrrh--equal portions;
gently massaged into the area being disturbed.
These should be alternated; not one used two
or three times and then the other two or three
times, but each day alternate; using the Camphorated Oil one time, the combination of Olive
Oil and Tincture Of Myrrh the next time, see?"*
1224-5

Peanut Oil massage:

*"Daily, for at least half to an hour and a half,
massage the body; not rudely, not crudely, not
with the attempt to make adjustments--for many
weeks yet. Massage with Peanut Oil--yes, the
lowly Peanut Oil has in its combination that
which will aid in creating in the superficial
circulation, and in the superficial structural
forces, as well as in the skin and blood, those
influences that make more pliable the skin,
muscles, nerves and tendons, that go to make
up the assistance to structural portions of
the body. Its absorption and its radiation
through the body will also strengthen the
activities of the structural body itself."*
2968-1

"In those areas from the 9th dorsal downward,
we find suppressions, subluxations and segments that have become static. Over these areas
we would apply, once or twice a week, oil heat
--as from toweling dipped in Peanut Oil and
applied with heat to the spinal area. Just
after these have been applied, have osteopathic adjustments made.
"Do this for 3 or 4 weeks, then leave off two
weeks, and then repeat. Keep this procedure
up for quite a long period, some 6 to 8 months
and we would find--with these general correc-
tions--there should be brought much better
conditions for this body." 4008-1

"...have every other day, at least, a deep
thorough massage along the spine with Peanut
Oil; then at times--at least once a week--with
an equal combination of Peanut Oil and Oil of
Pine Needles. But every other day in the evening
have a thorough massage with the Peanut Oil."
                                                    263-16
Peanut Oil and Olive Oil massage:

"After the massage, each time, we find it would
be well to massage the affected area--that
is--of course, across the small of the back
and extending all the way over the prostrate
area, you see, and on either side of the limbs
--with an equal combination of Olive Oil and
Peanut Oil. Massage in all the body will absorb. Do this after the manipulations are
given, each time." 1539-4

"About twice each week, almost bathe in Olive
Oil or Peanut Oil; especially Peanut Oil--in
the joints, the neck, across the clavicle,
across all areas of the spine, the rib and the
frontal area to the pit of the stomach, across
the stomach and especially in the diaphram
area; then across the hips and the lower portion
of the back and across the sacral area and
then the limb themselves." 1688-7

Salt and Apple Vinegar massage:

"The next day we would use the Salt (plain sodium chloride; not that carrying other properties, but this well powdered) and pure Apple Vinegar.
"Use one one day, the other the next day. Continue in this manner, and we find that these ingredients will supply calcium, acids and oils that will prevent accumulations of water...or prevent the tendons becoming so taut as not to allow movement in the knee and the kneecap."
438-5

These are but a minute samplings from the Cayce readings, and are each given for a specific purpose. The subject matter is too extensive to cover here but its importance is justified by the many recommendations found in the readings. This is a study in itself.

HYDROTHERAPY

PHYSIOLOGICAL EFFECT OF COLD AND HEAT

To understand the real relations that the ther-
mometric and barometric changes of the atmosphere
bear to the system, would relieve men of much of the
anxiety they habitually experience in regards to their
effects upon the health. Invalids, especially, are fond
of ascribing their depressed spirits to the state of
the weather, and very often attempt to get rid of a
disagreeable sense of personal responsibility by so
persuading themselves that their symptoms are attrib-
utable to some uncontrollable atmospheric cause. This
is convenient; but I am persuaded that a correct understanding of the intentions of nature toward us are
in these changes leading us to regard them, although
severe and untoward as they seem to us. When we unfit
ourselves sedulously from their effects, though most
friendly towards us and wisely and mercifully adapted
to maintain health, we suffer the consequences.

The average temperature of the air in this local
climate is not far from 55° Fahr.--the temperature of
our bodies is 98°; hence the average difference between
the heat of the body, and that of surrounding things
is not far from 43°; but the thermometer sometimes
falls considerably below zero, effecting a great
increase of this difference, from which it is apparent
that it is the intention of nature that the animal
body should be subjected not only by a high or a low,
but to a variable temperature. It is the nature of
heat or cold to be forever seeking an equilibrium, a
balance between its extremes.

Hence all bodies, whether animate or inanimate,
having a temperature above that of the atmosphere,
soon lose their excess, unless constantly replenished.
The rapidity with which an object loses heat depends
on the amount of difference between its temperature
and that of contiguous objects. But the living animal
body loses more heat in a given time period than an
inanimate body of the same size, weight, and warmth, for
it not only, like the stone, parts with its heat by

radiation to surrounding things, and by contact with them, but laso in ways peculiar to itself. The surface of the animal body is always moist, and evaporation from it is a most potent cooling agent. The body also parts with its heat through the action of several excretory organs, and a great deal is carried off by the large body of air which is constantly being warmed in the lungs.

The loss of heat which the body is thus compelled to sustain is perpetual, but is exceedingly variable in degree. The temperature of the atmosphere not only has its yearly and daily, its regular, and therefore its expected vicissitudes, but it is also subject to hourly and unexpected ones. We never know that the temperature will not rise or fall in a few hours by a number of degrees above or below the average point for the season. This uncertainty and variableness of temperature obtains to a greater degree or a lesser degree in all climates, which may be considered as ordained by the Creator for the benefit of all of his creatures; and thus may suppose that a uniformity of temperature would, contrary to the usual opinions of the invalid, be prejudicial to health.

Let us now look to the arrangements of the human system with reference to temperature, that we may the more easily understand those hygienic principles that relate thereto.

All atmospheric changes so impress the system as to modify its vital and its vito-chemical actions. All parts of the body are pervaded by sensory nerves, which receive such impressions and convey them in every direction. When the surface of the body, or any portion of it, receives an impression of external temperature, every part of the organism related to it in any way is immediately affected by it.

That function of the body which is most directly related to external impressions of temperature, is the heat-making process. The point of temperature at which vital actions take place being fixed, and the body heat being dependent upon its own resources, so it follows that the production of heat is accelerated or retarded to an extent exactly proportionate to the loss expe-

rienced--the process undergoing an amount of variation
just about equal to that which the sensory system is
subjected.

This regulation of the bodily temperature is
connected with the employment of the materials which
are necessary to the production of vital phenomena.
The system is thus relieved of any surplus of heat
which it may have acquired by means of an increased
evaporation from the surface, while the want of heat
that is felt stimulates the respiratory organs to
greater activity. Thus it appears that impressions
from without are as sure to affect the production of
heat, either to lessen or to augment it, as pressure
upon the key of the piano elicits a musical sound.
The slighest observation verifies these statements.
To place the hand, or foot, or any portion of the warm
surface of the person, in contact with a very cold
substance, as a piece of ice, instantaneously causes
an expansion of the ribs and a depression of the
diaphram, and consequently an unusually profound
inspiration, which is involuntary continued till the
heat that is thus lost is fully restored. The heat
of the body, or of any part, may for a short period
be depressed without injury, because it requires time
for the physiological changes now described to complete
their effects upon the economy. No artificiality of
heat is required in order to healthfully maintain the
bodily temperature; and when, by our fine civilized
modes of life we depress the heat-producing operations
of the body, we must remember that at the same time
we are impairing the respiratory acts, and are doing
ourselves more or less harm in proportion to the extent
of our misbehavior in this respect.

We may now understand some of the consequences
of inattention to the relations borne by the system
to temperature control in hot weather, and in hot
climates, the respiratory stimulus being less, respiration is consequently diminished, and thus results
in a retention of the materials that should be excluded
from the system through this agency. Such materials
are not completely reduced to carbonic acid water and
urea, but the process is arrested at an intermediate

point, and the state popularly termed biliousness,
which implies the presence in the blood of the prox-
imate elements of bile, inevitably succeeds, as unless
the person so exposed becomes very cautious as to his
diet and mental activities.

IMPORTANCE OF COLD

Chronic invalids are generally the victims of
the falsest notions respecting temperature. They have
become, by long habits of effeminacy, incapable of
bearing the amount of cold fitted to the respiratory
needs of the body. They exhibit the greatest suspicions
and fears of the most beneficent designs of nature.
They shrink from the very influence which elicits and
vivifies their powers, and so they continue to repress
and cramp their already weakened faculties. The importance of developing to a suitable and healthy extent
the heat-making faculty, is equal to that of exercise
and is among the first things to which the attention
of the chronic invalid should be directed.

The propriety of subjecting the system to the
influence of cold is not always to be decided by the
sensations, for these, except in perfect health, are
not to be trusted unless corroborated by the other
faculties. The effect of cold is to infuse into the
system an agreeable vigor and elasticity; but in a
weakened state of the system and perverted condition
of the nerves, the sensations, being abnormally acute,
will often rebel. This indicates the need for discipline, the very process required to reinstate health.
It is only under circumstances when the withdrawal of
heat from the system is not attended with a corresponding increase of respiration that exposure to cold
can be in any degree hurtful; for it is only then that
the refuse matter of the system is retained to be
subjected to that spontaneous chemical action which
will of course conflict with the vital processes.

Therefore, the treatment of acute diseases with
ice packs and cold ablutions is to promote the radiation of heat and thereby reduce the fever temperature,
the aim in the treatment of chronic diseases is to

arouse the system to acute eliminative effort. In other words, while the acute disease in hydropathic treatment is sedative, in chronic diseases it is just the opposite, it is stimulative.

WHY COLD WATER APPLICATIONS

1.- Stimulation of the Circulation: As stated before, cold water applied to the surface of the body arouses and stimulates the circulation all over the system. Blood counts before and after a cold-water application shows a marked increase in the number of red and white blood corpuscles. This does not mean that the cold water has in a moment created new blood cells, but it means that the blood has been stirred up and sent hurrying through the system, that those lazy blood cells which were lying inactively in the sluggish and stagnant blood stream and in the clogged and obstructed tissues are aroused to increased activity.

Undoubtedly, the invigorating and stimulating influence of cold water sprays, ablutions, sitzbaths, barefoot walking in the dewy grass or on wet stones, and all other cold-water applications depends largely upon their electro-magnetic effects upon the system.
2.- Eliminations of Impurities: As the cold water drives the blood with increased force through the system, it flushes the capillaries in the tissues and cleanses them from the accumulations of morbid matter and poisons which are one of the primary causes of acute and chronic diseases.

As the blood rushes back to the surface it suffuses the skin, opens and relaxes the pores and the minute blood vessels or capillaries, and thus unloads the impurities from the skin.

Hydrotherapy is a medical practice of extensive reputation, for its empirical success has been founded upon the use of temperature as a remedial means. Hydrotherapy, although a special, is a legitimate practice, because it is based on important, though not perhaps as practiced in sufficient numbers, the plain principles of physiology. The practice does consists of causing an artificial demand to be laid upon the system, or some limited portions of it, to produce heat, and also in repressing the natural production of heat in various parts by withdrawing the incentive thereto. In this way the most important changes may be induced in the circulation, the innervation, and nutrition of the various portions of the body, often sufficient, when skillfully managed, to restore the harmony and health of the organism.

In this practice, water, instead of air, is so employed, because it furnishes the means of applying temperature changes quickly, vigorouly, and extentsively, and is thus eminently adapted to meet most all emergencies of sickness, especially of acute disease. In bathing, it is the temperature of the water, rather than the water itself, which is to be regarded as the source of the effects which we often realize by the operation.

> "We would take, systematically, a series of hydrotherapy treatments. Each treatment should include a dry heat bath followed by the fumes with same of Witch Hazel; then the hot and cold shower, or needle shower; then the thorough rub down--a massage of the body with Pine Oil (preferably for this body)." 3000-1

COLD WATER FAVORED

In the treatment of chronic diseases some advocates of the natural methods of health prefer warm or hot applications in the form of hot water baths, of different kinds of steam or sweat baths, heat lamps, hot compresses, fomentation, etc.

However, the great majority of natural healing practioners in some countries have abandoned the hot applications of every kind almost entirely because of their weakening and enervating after-effects and because in many instances they have not only failed to produce the expected results, but aggravated the disease conditions.

However, the different effects of hot and cold water as well as all of the other therapeutic agents

upon the system can be explained by the law of action
and reaction.

Applied to physics, this law reads: "Action and
reaction are equal but opposite." The law of action
and reaction adapted to therapeutics in a somewhat
circumscribed manner follows: "Every therapeutic agent
affecting the human organism has a primary, TEMPORARY,
and secondary, PERMANENT effect. The secondary lasting
effect is contrary to the primary, transient effect."

The first, temporary effect of warmth above the
body temperature whether it be applied in the form of
hot air or water, steam, or light, is to draw the blood
to the surface. Immediately after such an application
the skin will be red and flushed.

The secondary and lasting effect, however, (in
accordance with the law of action and reaction) makes
the blood recedes into the interior of the body and
leaves the skin in a bloodless and enervated condition, subject to chills and predisposed to catching
colds as well as other complications.

On the other hand, the first, transient effect
of cold water application upon the body as a whole or
any particular part, is to chill the surface and send
the blood scurrying inward, leaving the skin in a
chilled, bloodless condition. This lack of blood and
sensation of cold are at once telegraphed over the
efferent nerves to headquarters in the brain, and from
there the command goes forth to the nerve centers regu-
lating the circulation: "Send blood to the surface."

As a result, the circulation is stirred up and
accelerated throughout the system, and the blood rushes
with force into the depleted skin, flushing the surface
of the body with warm, red blood, and restoring to it
the rosy color of health. This is the secondary effect.
In other words, the well-applied cold-water treatment
is followed by a good reaction, and this is accompanied
by many permanent beneficial results.

The drawing and eliminating primary effect of hot
applications, of sweat baths, etc., is at best only
temporary, lasting only a few minutes, and is always
followed by a weakening reaction, while the drawing
and eliminating action of the cold-water applications,

being the secondary, lasting effect, exerts an endur-
ing, invigorating, and tonic influence upon the skin
which enables it to throw off drosses not merely for
ten to fifteen minutes, as in the sweat bath under the
influence of excessive heat, but always, day or night.

THE MORNING COLD RUB

The essentials for a cold rub, and in fact for
every cold-water treatment, are warmth of the body
before the application, coolness of the water (natural
temperature), rapidity of action, and friction or
exercise to stimulate the circulation. No cold water
treatment should be taken when the body is in a chilled
condition.

Directly from the warmth of the bed, or after
sun bath and exercise have produced a pleasant glow
go to the bathroom, sit in the empty tub with the
stopper in place, turn on the cold water, and as it
flows into the tub, catch it in the hollow of the hands
and wash first the limbs, then the abdomen, then chest
and back. Throw the water all over the body and rub
the skin with the hands as when you wash your face.

Do this quickly but thoroughly. The entire procedure need not take up more than a few minutes. By the
time the bath is finished, there may be from two to
four inches of water in the tub. Use a towel or brush
for the back if you cannot reach it otherwise.

As long as there is a good reaction, the cold rub
may be taken in an unheated bathroom even in coldest
of weather.

After the bath, dry the body quickly with a coarse
towel and finish by rubbing with the hands until the
skin is dry and smooth and you are aglow with the
exercise, or expose the wet body to the fresh air
before an open window and rub with the hands until dry
and quite warm.

A bath taken in this manner combines the beneficial
effects of cold water, air, exercise, and the magnetic
friction of the hands on the body. No lifeless instruments or mechanical appliance can ever be equal to the
dexterity, warmth, and magnetism of the human hand.

The bath must be so conducted that it is followed by a feeling of warmth and comfort. Some persons will be benefited by additional exercise, or better still, a brisk walk in the open air, while others will get better results by returning to the warmth of the bed.

There is no better means for stimulating the general circulation and for increasing the eliminative activities of the system than this cold morning rub at the beginning of the day, after a good night's rest. If this is kept up regularly, its good effects will soon become apparent.

This method of taking a morning bath is to be preferred to the plunge into a tub filled with cold water. While persons with very strong constitutions may experience no ill effects, to those who are weak and who do react readily, the cold plunge might prove a severe shock and strain upon the system.

When a bathtub is not available, take the morning cold rub in the following manner:

Stand in an empty washtub. In front of you place a basin or bucket filled with cold water. Wet the hands or a towel and wash the body, part by part, from the feet upward, then dry and rub with the hands as previously directed.

> "Use water inside and outside for the body. Keep the system cleansed, for this will allow the perfect assimilation and the perfect eliminations, with the body set in its proper vibration. In applying the water externally, would be to produce all along the nerve centers of the cerebro-spinal system, each morning, COLD, see? and rubbed until the body is aglow, as it were, for each center then receives its proper stimulation, and the whole vibration will be set in better attunement." 121-1

EFFECT ON THE NERVES

It will be noticed that temperature, especially a low degree of it, acts primarily upon the nerves and, also it is thought the intervention of these has its effects upon the circulation, respiration, nutrition, etc., are chiefly wrought. The great majority of people, whose sensory surface is too little exposed are greatly benefited by the stimulation and vigorous tone that is afforded by the daily morning bath and rub. It counteracts in the sedentary the ill effects of warm air confined next to the person by clothing, and for all who are not constantly out of doors, it is an important means for maintaining the health. But serious ill effects may, and very frequently do, arise from too much, and injudicious bathing. The abuse here alluded to arise from an ignoring of the principles relating to the harmony of function, insisted on in this volume. It will be understood that all impressions made upon external sensory nerves are accompanied by corresponding action of the nerve-centers situated in the brain, spinal cord, and especially those of the trunk, as the seat of the nerves of organic life. Stimulant impressions, if habitually resorted to, induce hypernutrition, and consequently excite an unbalanced action of the nervous system, which is utterly incompatible with health. Persons who, for a length of time, so subject themselves frequently to repeated and intense impressions of heat and cold, by means of water bathing, abuse themselves in a way that will certainly be followed by irregular nervous action, and the various grades of nervous disease-- excitability, depression of spirits, neuralgia, hypochondria, etc. Great caution should be used that this mode of healthful stimulation be not made a substitute for the more common nerve stimulants which proper hygiene condemns. The water-cure, so called at times, is somewhat practiced more to the detriment than to the benefit of individuals.

COLD WATER APPLICATION

The duration of the cold-water applications must be regulated by the individual conditions of the person and by his powers of reaction; but it should be borne in mind that it is the short and the quick application that produces the stimulating, electro-magnetic effects upon the system. The temperature of the water should range from 40-55 degrees, and that its duration is about one and a half minutes to three minutes time periods. It is refreshing to the nerves, stimulating to the heart rate, and increasing respiration and metabolism activity.

By far the largest number of deaths in febrile diseases result from the accumulation in the system of poisonous substances, which paralyzes or destroys vital centers and organs. Therefore, it is necessary to eliminate the morbid products of inflammation from the organism as quickly as possible.

This also is accompanied most effectively, and thoroughly, by the application of wet packs. As they draw the blood into the surface and relax the minute blood vessels in the skin, the morbid materials in the blood are eliminated through the pores of the skin and absorbed by the packs. That this is actually so, is verified by the yellowish or brownish discolorations of the wet wrappings and by their offensive odors.

EVENING COLD SITZ BATH

The morning cold rub is stimulating in its effects, the evening sitz bath is quieting and relaxing. The latter is therefore especially beneficial if taken just before going to bed.

The cold water draws the blood from brain and spinal cord and thereby insures better rest and sleep. It cools and relaxes the abdominal organs, sphincters, and orifices, stimulates gently and naturally the action of the bowels and of the uninary tract, and is equally effective in chronic constipation and in the affections of the kidneys or bladder.

The sitz bath is best taken in the regular sitz bathtub made for the purpose, but an ordinary bathtub, or washtub or large pan may be used with equally good effect.

Pour into the vessel a few inches of water at natural temperature, as it comes from the faucet, and sit in the water unto a good reaction takes place-- that is, until the first sensation of cold is followed

by a feeling of warmth. This may take, from a few
seconds to a few minutes, according to the temperature
of the water and the individual powers of reaction.

Dry with a coarse towel, rub and pat the skin
with the hands, then, in order to establish a good
reaction, practice deep breathing for a few minutes,
alternating with the head and neck exercises.

In acute disease water treatment will accomplish
all of the beneficial effects by which the old school
practitioners ascribe to drugs, and it will therefore
produce the desired results much more efficiently and
without any harmful effects or after effects upon the
system.

The principal objectives to be attained in the
treatment of acute inflammatory diseases are:
1.- To relieve the inner congestion and consequent
pain in the affected parts.
2.- To keep the temperature below the danger point
by promoting heat radiation through the skin.
3.- To increase the activity of the organs of elimination and thus to facilitate the removal of morbid
materials from the system.
4.- To increase the positive electro-magnetic energies in the organism.
5.- To increase the amount of oxygen and ozone in
the system and thereby promote the oxidation and the
combustion of effete matter.

The above mentioned objects can be attained most
effectually by the simple cold water treatment. Whatever the acute condition may be, whether an ordinary
cold or the most serious type of febrile disease. The
applications described, used singly, or combined, or
alternately according to individual conditions, will
always be in order and sufficient to produce the best
possible results.

THE WARM BATH

When the temperature of the air is considerably
below that of the body, we know that it receives heat
from it at only very low rates; but water does not
feel warm to us until its temperature approximates

very nearly our own. At 98° it ceases to receive heat
from us, and therefore, when the body is submerged in
a bath of that temperarure, the ordinary incentive to
the production of heat ceases to act, and the physiological processes are retarded, respiration becomes
slow and difficult, and the system soon suffers from
retained matters. If there has been pain, the bath
affords oftentimes a delightful sense of relief, and
frequently checks morbid action. These efforts become
less apparent at slightly lower temperatures; and when
still further reduced, the effects as experienced are
those of the cold bath to a moderate degree.

The reader will note an important and radical
difference between the effects of cold and those of
warm bathing. Cold baths, on account of their effects
on respiration, are an agency for the removal from the
body of its solid materials; while warm and hot baths,
by the effort assist the system in making to relieve
itself of heat, remove the fluid and saline matters,
therefrom. In many cases of disease both agents, hot
or cold, are required of these.

HOW TO KEEP THE FEET WARM

The proverb says: "Keep the head cool and the
feet warm."This is good advice, but most people try
to follow it by doctoring their cold feet with hot
water bottles, warming pads, hot bricks, etc., These
are excellent means of making the feet still colder,
because heat makes cold and cold makes heat.

In accordance with the law of action and reaction,
hot applications drive the blood away from the feet
while cold applications draw the blood to the feet.
Therefore, if your feet are cold and bloodless (which
means that the blood is congested in other parts of
the body), walk barefoot in the dewy grass, in a cool
brook, on wet stone pavements, or on the snow.

Instead of putting a hot water bottle to the feet
of a bed-ridden invalid, bathe his feet with cold water
adding a little salt for its electric effect, then rub
and knead (massage), and then finish with a magnetic
treatment by holding the feet between your hands and

willing the blood to flow into them. This will have a
lasting effect not only upon the feet, but upon the
entire organism.

The application of the bath to a limited portion
of the body is governed by the same general principles
as govern its application to the whole surface. But
the response made by the system to the impression of
the local bath is peculiar. If the bath is cold, the
process causes the heat of the body to depart from it
through a circumscribed surface. Now, since the heat
is applied to the cold part affecting the blood as it
flows thitherward, the process of local bathing then
becomes one of calling, or deriving the circulation
from the general system in the direction of the cold
part. This effect is eminently useful in aiding similar
effects produced by movements for the removal of morbid
matter and visceral congestion.

THE HOT BATH

In a bath of this sort, heat is imparted to the
body, the effect of which is to compel it to take on
a reciprocal action and return of what it has received,
by producing moisture on the surface, to be evaporated.
The skin, under the influence of the hot bath, breaks
out in a copious perspiration, this effect following
with a rapidity proportioned to the temperature. When
this effect is produced, the superficial capillaries
are filled with blood, and central portions of the body
consequently relieved from their engorgement, often,
especially in severe internal congestion, to the temporary relief of the complaint. The effect described
here can not be long continued, for obvious reasons,
without serious detriment to the entire organism.

HOT SITZ BATH

The hot sitz bath has numerous benefits and uses.
It is chiefly used for warming and relaxing the body,
especially before retiring. However, if the body is
rather on the cool side to take a cold sitz bath, it
can be used to warm up the body before taking the cold

one. The hot sitz bath helps to relieve the discom-
forts of rectal complications and disorders.

SWEAT CABINET BATH

The sweat cabinet bath is extensively explained
in the Cayce readings and was recommended for many
different ailments.

> *"Eliminations are the cause of the disorder
> in the lower portions of the system (feet,
> ankles and limbs)--as well as producing a
> tendency for portions of the body especially--
> to be out of proportion to the body as a whole.
> "These conditions may be aided most if the
> body were to be more mindful of the diet. Not
> as an extremist, no, but a diet that would make
> corrections in the general eliminating system.
> "This would be an outline for the correction
> of the physical conditions that may later
> produce hindrances in the general physical
> health of the body.
> "We would begin first with those colonic
> irrigations--one every ten days until four or
> five are taken, which will overcome this
> tendency of constipation through the system.
> "We would also have at least twice each week,
> sweat cabinet baths, with a thorough rub down
> afterwards, using any of the eleminants, or
> prepare as this: Take Russian White Oil, one
> pint; alcohol, one pint; and Witch Hazel one-
> half pint. Mix these together and massage the
> body with same following the baths, see? Well
> to occasionally leave off the oil rub and use
> a salt glow--that is rub the body with salt."*
> *2096-1*
> *"After the four osteopathic adjustments have
> been given, begin with the hydrotherapy treat-
> ments. These would include sweats, though do
> not have the temperature too high in the dry
> cabinet. Preferably have some fume bath with
> same--using Witch Hazel in the fume. Use the*

*fume inside the dry cabinet, you see, by
putting a tablespoonful of Witch Hazel in half
a pint of water and letting it boil as in a
croup cup; letting the steam from same settle
over the body in the closed cabinet, see?*
*"Then have a thorough massage and rubdown
following the sweat, to stimulate the circulation; and especially in the massage use an
equal combination of Olive Oil and Peanut Oil,
for the heavy veins on limbs and the irritation
to the superficial circulation--for the increasing of better eliminations.*
*"These sweats and massages we would take at
least once a week (after they are begun) until
at least five have been taken.*
*"During that period there would be given at
least one colonic irrigation, preferably after
the first sweat or massage--after there has
been the taking of the compound indicated for
purification of alimentary canal--that is, the
Sulphur compound, see?"* 2455-1

*"We would find first, then, that there should
be the use of the sweat baths; those that carry
not a raising of the temperature of the body
to a great extent...but rather FUME baths,
where there is used in same an alternation of
Oil of Wintergreen and the Tincture of Iodine
--or that of Atomidine full strength; one used
one day of the treatment, the other at the
next treatment...with the thorough rubdown
after same."* 1302-1

*"We would have prepared a cabinet or a canvas
covering in which sweats may be taken. In same
put the fumes of Witch Hazel; at least an ounce,
to an ounce and a half in about four ounces of
water that would be boiled in the cabinet...
Take such a fume bath, or cabinet sweat, every
other day; followed with a thorough rubdown
...all the body will absorb of Peanut Oil,
mixing just enough Olive Oil (commercial oil*

> *will do) to prevent irritation. Pour the oil*
> *into a saucer, dipping the fingers or hands*
> *in same to massage the body." 2526-1*

EPSOM SALTS TREATMENT

The use of Epsom Salts internally and externally, is in harmony with the natural therapeutics in so far as the alkaline magnesium tends to neutralize and to eliminate negative pathogenic substances, such as carbon and nitrogen compounds, from the system. While Epsom Salts taken internally as a laxative, or externally in the form of baths, packs and compresses, is a very powerful neutralizer and eliminator of acids, ptomaines and xanthins, we must not overlook the fact that the inorganic minerals it contains have a strong tendency to accumulate in the system and to form many deposits which may in time become as harmful as the morbid materials which the salts are meant to eliminate from the system.

Epsom Salts baths, packs and compresses are very useful in cases of acute inflammatory rheumatism, gout, pneumonia, Bright's disease, appendicitis, ptomaine poisoning and in all other feverish diseases, but under no circumstances is it recommended to use the salt for long continued treatment.

The therapeutic action of Epsom Baths consists in stimulating the eliminative activity of the skin, its pores and glandular structures. This result is also contained in a lesser degree by ordinary table salt and by sea salt.

The Epsom Salts may be applied to the skin in warm or cold solutions, in the form of local applications in wet packs or compresses, as a general sponge bath, the whole body or as a sitz or hip bath.

> *"We would have every day at least one bath*
> *with a good amount of Epsom Salts in it,*
> *following this with a good rubdown along the*
> *whole cerebro-spinal system.*
> *"The Epsom Salts baths would be taken during*
> *the day. Put a pound of salts to about ten to*

*twenty gallons of water; not too hot but
rather a tepid bath, but remain in same so
that the absorption and reaction to the whole
nerve system is received. Add a little hot
water to keep this warm...from 20 to 30 minutes.
"Have this about once each week...Use about
ten lbs. of Epsom Salts in about 40 gallons
of water, and this pretty warm...for 3 weeks
...(omit) for 6 weeks, another, then, would
be taken but increase the amount of Epsom
Salts to 15 pounds. Massage over spine during
the bath. After, massage with Peanut Oil."*

                                        5169-1

*"There are changes in the physical forces of
the body, as is indicated by the better use
of the limbs, of the changes in the eliminations and in the distribution of that as is
assimilated. In the releasing of the pressures
as have been apparent in the lumbar, the
sacral, and especially the coccyx, we will
find that nerve energy to extremities will be
more active in its activities in the physical
functioning of the body.
"It would be well that there be added the
saturated solutions or packs of Epsom Salts,
and that the stimulation, after the manipulative measures in lumbar and sacral—be through
the applying of the violet ray, rather than
the ultra violet." 53-2*

*"Q.- Do you advise the use of colonics or Epsom
Salts baths for this body?
"A.- When these are necessary, yes. For everyone, every body, should take an internal bath
occasionally, as well as an external one. They
would all be better off if they would."440-3*

Edgar Cayce recommended Epsom Salts baths for a
variety of sicknesses. The following readings bring
forth the variations as well as the purposes for the
treatments. They are excellent for releasing morbid
matter from the entire system.

"*Conditions as we find are very good in many respects, but those tendencies for the accumulations--or crystalization of the activities through the system, from the lack of lymph flow--are still indicated at times; in the joints of the fingers, in the wrist and hand, and at times in the ankles, or the extremities --the superficial and deeper circulation.*
"*The better means of keeping these in check is the use of the Epsom Salts bath at least once a month, oftener if there is more trouble caused. Fill the tub as full as you can with water, body-temperature, with at least five to ten pounds of Epsom Salts dissolved in same. Lie in this. Add the hot water if necessary, after lying in same for a time. Stay in this for at least twenty to thirty minutes, during this period massage those areas affected.*
"*Then, if there is particular pain in the joints, use the Epsom Salts Packs--such as on the fingers or wrist or the like; a saturated solution of Epsom Salts, hot.*
"*Follow each of these-whether the bath or the Packs--with a Peanut Oil rub.*" 340-44

"*As we find, there is a tendency in the body for the crystallization of acids that have been a part of the condition in the system from toxic forces.*
"*Then--at least once in two weeks, or once every ten days until five or six are taken, we would take an Epsom Salts Bath. Have an almost saturated solution; that is, fill the tub with water as hot as the body can well stand, and stir in same about eight pounds of Epsom Salts. Lie in this for at least thirty minutes; gradually massaging the joints in the lower limbs, joints in the hands and arms and shoulders with the solution while in the bath.*
"*Sponge off thoroughly, and massage thoroughly with plain Peanut Oil (not other things added) --over the arms and shoulders and limbs, and*

across the hips.

"Do not do this too often, but do it at least about every ten days for the first three to four times; then it may be done once a month or the like....

"Q.- Why do I sleep so restlessly even tho I'm tired?

"A.- Pressure upon the nerves of the joints by the crystallization of acids in the system. The Baths and Rubs as indicated should eliminate this entirely from the system, taken in time and being persistent." 340-43

One of the most beneficial applications consists in sponging the entire body with a solution of Epsom Salts for a period of from five to ten minutes and then going to bed without drying. This draws the blood into the cuticle, makes the skin more alive and active as it opens the pores and draws the pathogenic matter to the surface. It acts as a powerful stimulant to the glandular structures of the skin, promotes elimination and relieves the poisoned and overburdened heart and other vital organs. In similar manner it relieves the heat-regulating center in the medulla and thereby reduces the temperature in febrile conditions.

Undoubtedly a great part of the beneficial effect is due to the action of the water itself in the ablutions and compresses. The Epsom Salt solution may be applied also in the form of cooling hip or sitz baths, or in the natural bath. In all cases the Epsom Salts will heighten the tonic effect of the water.

The continued use of the salt is not recommended in such applications because the cold water alone, used continuously in the form of tonic applications, is powerful enough to suffice for the requirements of the various regimen in health and disease. In acute febrile conditions, however, when rapid neutralization and elimination of pathogenic materials becomes imperative, tonic applications of sea salt and Epsom Salts will be found very beneficial.

ENEMAS AND COLONICS FLUSHINGS

Injections of warm water into the rectum are taken
in order to relieve the constipated intestines of
accumulation of fecal material and thus to prevent the
re-absorption of morbid matter and systemic poisons.

The necessity for enemas or colonics is a sure sign
that the person who needs them has not been living the
natural life. If he had, he would not be constipated.

The only way to restore the natural activity of
the bowels in cases of chronic constipation is through
natural diet, fasting when indicated, and through the
use of suitable additions of bulk to the diet.

There is much on this subject in the readings.

*"Take a colonic irrigation occasionally, or
have one administered, scientifically. One
colonic irrigation will be worth about four
to six enemas."* 3570-1

*"Some disturbances are indicated in the diges-
tive forces of the body. These are from the
lack or proper eliminations even though there
are regularities...the eliminations need to be
increased from these angles. This may be done
in no better manner than by having colonic
irrigations occasionally and by including in
the diet such things as figs, rhubarb and the
like."* 4003-1

*"As indicated--see--there are channels or
outlets for the eliminating of poisons; that
is, used energies, where there is the effect
of the activity of the circulation upon foreign
forces...These all, by the segregating of same
in the system, produce forces which are to be
eliminated. We eliminate principally through
the activity of the lungs, of course, and the
perspiratory system, the alimentary canal and
the kidneys...The head aches are the signs
or warnings that eliminations are not being
properly cared for. Most of this, in this body,*

*comes from the alimentary canal, and from those
conditions that exists in portions of the colon
itself, as to produce a pressure upon (these)
...Hence the suggestion for the osteopathic
corrections, which aid but which do not eliminate all of those conditions which are as
accumulations through portions of the colon.
Consequently, colonic irrigations are necessary, occasionally, as well as general hydrotherapy and massage."* 2602-2

Therefore:

*"Every one—everybody--should take an internal
bath occasionally as well as an external one.
They would all be better off if they would."*
                                        440-3

The use of enemas and colonics is recommended in
the Edgar Cayce readings for the treatment of certain
disease, during fasting, and in stubborn constipation
cases, or by "everybody" according to the readings
above, yet the word utilized is "occasionally." These
taken habitually have a weakening effect upon the
intestines. As the saying goes, they make them "more
lazy." The reason for this is obvious. Dryness of the
fecal matter is the stimulus for the secretion of those
mucous fluids by the membranous linings of the bowels.
When the intestines are constantly flooded with water
injected through the rectum, the stimulus to secretion
is lacking and the cellular linings and glandular
structures of the intestines become more inactive. Any
function of the organism which we do not use on a
regular basis, atrophies.

Continued flooding with warm water has a very
relaxing effect upon the intestines. The tone of the
muscular tissues is lowered from day to day and the
intestines become distended, forming pockets for the
retention of putrefying fecal matter. Like drugs and
laxatives, the internal bath in the long run creates
the very condition which it is supposed to cure,
namely, greater inactivity and atrophy. However, the
choice remains, which is dependent on our condition.

"Q.- How often should hydrotherapy be given?
"A.- Dependent upon the general conditions.
Whenever there is a sluggishness, the feeling
of heaviness, oversleepiness, the tendency for
an achy, draggy feeling, then have the treat-
ments. This does not mean that merely because
there is the daily activity of the alimentary
canal there is not the need for flushing the
system. But whenever there is the feeling of
slugginess have the treatments. It'll pick the
body up. For there is a need for such treat-
ments when the condition of the body becomes
drugged because of the absorption of poisons
through alimentary canal or colon, slugginess
of liver or kidneys, and there is the lack
of co rdination with the cerebro-spinal and
sympathetic, blood supply and nerves. For the
hydrotherapy and massage are preventative as
well as curative measures. For the cleansing
of the system allows the body's forces them-
selves to function normally, and thus eliminate
poisons, or congestions and conditions that
should become acute through the body."

                                        257-254

In all acute, inflammatory febrile diseases enemas
are given in the beginning, daily, and after that at
longer intervals, according to the nature of the case
and the vitality of the patient. Fasting in acute
disease and increased heat in the abdominal organs
usually produce constipation. We can overcome this
difficulty by enemas. This empties the lower intestines
of morbid accumulations and prevents re-absorption of
poisonous secretions. The bowels should be emptied as
nearly as possible during the early stages of a fever,
as long as the vitality is unimpaired.

While fasting the bowels usually cease moving,
though there are some exceptions where the bowels keep
moving daily for a week or so although no food was
taken. If they cease to move soon after the fast is
entered upon, it is best to give enemas or colonics
in order to evacuate the intestines and so therefore
prevents the re-absorption of poisonous excretions.

"...Have a good hydrotherapist give a thorough but gentle colon cleansing....In the first waters, use salt and soda, in the proportions of a heaping teaspoonful of table salt and a level teaspoonful of baking soda dissolved thoroughly--to each half gallon of water. In the last use Glyco-Thymoline as an intestinal antiseptic to purify the system, in the proportions of a tablespoonful to the quart of water." 1745-4

"We would in the present begin, surely--gently, but each day--with tepid water high enemas, gradually dilating the lower portion of the colon and anus...It will be necessary that this be done gradually, but in a five day period the blood pressure should be reduced at least 30 or 40 points--or more. Begin as in this manner, with the water for the enema: "To three quarts of water add a level teaspoonful of salt and a heaping teaspoonful of baking soda.
"We would also use the oils in the last portion of the enema, that to remain in the bowel as much or as long as possible. The (last) quart of water we would use at least a heaping tablespoonful of the Petrolagar. Stir this thoroughly as it is injected." 381-2

"When there is the lack of eliminations through the alimentary canal, then to cleanse the colon, have the irrigation. Whether this is necessary once a week, twice a week, once in six weeks or once in six months depends upon the manner in which the body treats itself."
303-34
"But these are well to be used when needed. If they are given body temperature with the water used, and the cleansing solution in same, the Salt and Soda in proportions indicated, and the Glyco-Thymoline as the purifier or the like--these will not be weakening but will

*help. But too often given, too hot or too cold
water, they will be disturbing." 303-31*

*"...Give a colonic irrigation, using the high
tube; not just an ordinary tube, but a colon
tube, see? For this must empty the colon, so
that there will be a reaction of the peristaltic movement. In the first water use a
heaping teaspoonful of salt and a level teaspoonful of soda. In the last quart and a half
of water put a tablespoonful of Glyco-Thymoline." 1312-5*

However:

*"They (colonics) are seldom curative, unless
there are those measures taken to aid in correcting the cause of the disturbance." 303-34*

TREATMENT OF CONSTIPATION

The readings of Edgar Cayce state that the basis
of most disease was the internal uncleanliness. They so
regard eliminations through skin, lungs, kidneys and
intestines as secondary in importance only to correct
eating. Correct eating and adequate eliminations was
his basic formula for the treatment of most chronic
diseases.

The readings first attention was always directed
to the proper bowel action. Constipation was considered the fore-runner and producer of most of all the
troubles from which chronic cases suffered.

For 2000 years the men of medicine have tried to
solve the problem of constipation. Practically every
mineral and plant known to man has been tried, adopted
or discarded as the case might be. Herbs, drugs, and
minerals produced catharasis but did not cure constipation. Some 90 years ago the work of Dr. Graham, (the
inventor of graham crackers) opened the eyes of alert
physicians to the value of accessory foods, roughage,
bulk and lubricant foods, foods which would not be
digested but which would faithfully serve the purposes
of mechanical digestion.

"Mornings--At least twice to three times each week there should be taken that cracked wheat cereal or whole wheat; not oats, but that which is cooked in such a manner that the whole evaluation of the vitamins of the iron, silicon, the roughage as necessary for the creating of the proper balance in the blood supply, is effective to the body. There may be periods when fresh fruits may be taken in preference to either of these." 829-1

"Rather we would use the cereal combinations as of malt and the whole wheat, that would be better. These will supply malt in the digestive forces, with the weight, with the activities for all--especially with those properties as indicated that produce a cleansing that is hard to surpass." 1206-2

"The lacking for the system, then, is the body --or the weight, to make for the activities through the gastric flow of the digestive system: for these having been the first basis of disturbances, we must be precautious as to increasing this too fast or overbalancing in elements that would make for an infection--or a centralizing of poisons in the organs of assimilation.
"Hence we would begin with what may be termed some of the pre-digested foods, or whole wheat that is rolled and then cooked for two or two and a half hours--only, though, in enamel or glassware. While this carries a great deal of starch, it would be very strengthening and helpful if taken in moderation; that is, in small quantities at the time and given the more often--every hour or the like, you see, not more than a half to a teaspoonful at the time, and this taken slowly, with milk and a little brown sugar for the seasoning. This carries those balances of iron and the vitamin elements in phosphorous, the forces in silicon,

*and the activities necessary to make for a
complete balance in the body.*
*"So the beef juices and the whole wheat (this
rolled or crushed, not ground) should be sufficient for the next eight days, with—of
course—the fruits and vegetable juices that
have been indicated." 556-8*

Therefore:

Every meal needs in it some indigestible or pre-
digested substance which will produce "action" in the
intestines! The barnyard fowl eats gravel to get bulk
or weight for a stimulus to the intestinal tract. The
cat nibbles at blades of grass, as does the pet dog.
All animals use accessory foods. Only man has been
too busy and too civilized to adopt this natural means
of promoting elimination. So the introduction of a
balanced accessory food is one of nature's greatest
contribution to the health and welfare of mankind.
This fascinating fact of a bulk food which would be
palatable and could be added to the meal without great
trouble, and being comparatively inexpensive, would
wean mankind away from drugs, purgatives and the many
types of laxatives now on the market.
      To find a simple food additive to prevent cons-
tipation, a food laxative, not a drug laxative, is
ideal because a basic cause of constipation is wrong
eating. While purgatives or physics will forcibly expel
waste materials, they are not curative, but harmful.
They fail completely in the treatment of this disease
which saps the health and well-being and devitalizes
uncounted millions of sufferers.

*"Q.- Are any laxatives necessary; if so, what
special ones are best for me?*
*"A.- We are preparing the system so that these
will not be necessary! The laxatives will be
within those properties taken as the general
tonic, or for the toning of the system; with
the food values and the enemas, for the time
being!...Let's do this first, and then we may
ask more questions." 274-2*

Knowledge of the human body and how it works is a profound mystery for too many people. Let us consider now, in its simplest phases, the gigantic task which our digestive system performs in taking the foods we eat, digesting them, assimilating the nourishment which they contain and rejecting the waste. Why does it expell the poisonous matter from the body? why it does so, and what can be done about it.

Food passes from the stomach directly into the small intestines, where the process of digestion is continued. Millions of blood vessels in the intestinal wall carry the blood to this feeding ground, where the proteins, fats, sugars, starches, mineral salts, and all the nourishing ingredients of the foods we eat are absorbed by the blood and carried throughout the body. The remainder--waste--is carried along to the large intestines, or colon, where it is forced along upward through that part of the colon which commences at the lower right-hand side of the body, then across the body just below the stomach; then down the left-side, and on to the rectum where it is expelled.

The total distance of this journey covers well over thirty feet. Since this course is both tortuous and contrary to the force of gravity along some of its length, some other force must be exerted in this work of expelling the body' poisons. This force is called "Peristalsis." It is when your peristaltic action is faulty that you become constipated.

PERISTALSIS is the continuous waves of the muscles on the intestinal walls--a series of contractions which force the contents of the intestines onward. This muscular action is purely involuntary; nature intended the entire function to be performed without conscious effort on our part.

The only proper remedy for constipation is the one which stimulates normal, natural peristalsis. Laxatives, physics, cathartics and similar drugs cannot do this. Some achieve their results by irritating the intestinal wall, causing a copious watering similar to that of the eye when a foreign substance enters. This water serves in carrying waste along with it and out of the body. Still others whip up the peristaltic

muscles to furious and unnatural activity in the manner
of stimulants. However, these muscles gradually become
accustomed to the action of these stimulants and so,
require larger and larger doses before there is any
further response. Finally they become so used to the
stimulants that they will not work well at all.

Obviously, these emergency measures, for that is
all that there are, do nothing to correct the condition
which causes constipation, and afford only a temporary
relief. In addition, because they tend to tear down
the intestinal system rather than to build it up, they
are highly destructive and dangerous.

Still another emergency measure which involves
unnatural stimulation is the enema, though recommended
in the readings, is not a cure of the problem. The
poisonous filth diluted by an enema, but none the less
poisonous, is carried high into the intestines, is
absorbed by the blood and eliminated from its accumulation in the colon only at the expense of sending it
widespread throughout the body. If you have ever had
occassion to observe the immediate after effects of
an enema, you will have noted that a headache becomes
perceptibly worse just after administering this treat-
ment--the result of this rapid spread of the poisons of
autointoxication throughout the system. Enemas are
also condemned because constant use tends to weaken
and eventually destroy the power of the muscular tissue
of the bowels. This is more or less put forth in the
following Cayce reading.

> *"These congestions caused in the trachea, the
> conditions in the heart activity--the pressure
> is near normal at most times. When there is
> over-exercise physically, or especially the
> mental forces as of worry or anxiety, to be
> sure it calls on the necessity of those emunc-
> tory activities--or those patches that are
> called by a man's name. These are then lessened
> in their number and thus make a quickening,
> or an anxiety, causing the flow of blood in
> the heart, as an organ, to dilate. In making
> administrations to supply those glandulars*

centers which supply to these patches, or the emunctories, add those in the B complex or the Riboflavin--the necessary elements in each portion of the B vitamon forces.

For: (continuing)

"...the excess use of salines to flush or to cleanse the colon has reduced in blood more of that which causes that plasm. Thus the inabilities of these centers, those patches through which there are the areas of the lymph circulation, are such as to cause ofttimes a state of disintegration. In these patches, then, there is a lack of sufficient globular forces to cause the coagulation in the flow of the lymph, or that portion of same which is the leucocyte, or the sticky portion in the blood is not sufficient to make perfect contact between sympathetic and cerebro-spinal activities of the body." 294-212

And:

"There is stil at times incoordination in the sympathetics through the activities to the cerebro-spinal and to the sensory reactions (we are speaking from the physical angle entirely in the present, you see), yet there has been created--by the activities of the properties in the system--more of a stimuli to the coordinating reactions, in the form of filaments of circulation through the activities of plasm, in the nerve forces themselves, as well as a better application of the blood supply about those portions through which the nerve plasm operates." 386-3

Therefore:

"As we find, unless there are measures taken the conditions here may become very serious.

These are the conditions as we find them with this body, (1836).

"There having been a disturbance in the lacteal ducts, there has been a disturbance that causes an adhesion in this portion of the body; and at times a drawing in the right side (right) just below the liver and the gall duct area.

"This disassociation causes a breakage in the coordinating of the cerebro-spinal and sympathetic nervous system, until there are the tendencies and impulses for an overflow of the nerve impulse through the cerebro-spinal system.

"And these, unless some measures are taken, may form a clot or a break in the brain.

"As to the general conditions of the body, these are gradually giving way to these disturbances--both from the physical reaction and from the anxiety in the self as well as those about the body.

"Then, as we find:

"We would apply, consistently, for at least ten such applications, the Castor Oil Packs-- about every other evening, when the body is ready to retire, for an hour; the Packs changed about twice during the hour period. These would be applied over the caecum and the gall duct area, or the right side from the ribs to the point of the hip, extending lower than the abdomen in that area, see? Use about three thicknesses of flannel, wrung out of the hot Castor Oil and applied, then a pad put over same, and then the electric pad or dry heat put over same to keep it warm or as hot as the body can stand it, see? Do this every other evening for at least TEN such applications, making a period of twenty days, see?

"Also, each evening, for at least twenty to thirty days, we would massage the spine--downward; beginning at the base of the brain; one day using OLIVE OIL, the next day using Cocoa Butter. Massage all the body will absorb. Let

this extend on either side of the spinal column
from the base of the brain to the end of the
spine; gently, in a rotary motion, massaged
into the body, see? Rub AWAY FROM the head,
always. Take about twenty to thirty minutes
each evening to give this massage, see?

"After the massage, as ALSO after the Castor
Oil Packs, the body may be sponged off--the
areas of the massage AND the Packs--with luke-
warm soda water if desired.

"In the diet--keep away from fried foods and
from any hog meat of ANY kind--especially
sausage and the like.

"Do these and as we find we may aid in eliminating these disturbances.

"Then, at the end of the twenty to thirty days
of following these directions, we would give
further directions.

"Ready for questions.

"Q.- Is this the cause for the curious spells
he has been having off and on for the last
six years?

"A.- This causes the spells--the losing of
consciousness and the like.

"We are through for the present." 1836-1

CASTOR OIL PACKS

"We find that the Castor Oil Packs over the
abdomen and right side would be well occasionally for the lack of eliminations. When these
ARE applied, and the general massage is given
following same, give a quantity of Olive Oil
--just so it is not sufficient to cause regurgitation or vomitting--we will find it will
work well with the assimilating, and act as
a food as well as an eliminant for the alimentary canal." 1553-7

"As we find, the acute conditions arise from
the effects of a poison--Pyrene. From this activity the acute indigestion produced through

the alimentary canal, has caused an expansion
of, and a blocking in the colon areas.
"As we find in the present, we would apply hot
Castor Oil Packs continually, for two and a
half to three hours. Then have an enema, gently
given...only oil given first, see? Olive Oil
would be better for this, about half a pint
--so that there may be the relaxing. And then
give the enema with body temperature water,
using a heaping teaspoonful of salt and a level
teaspoonful of baking soda to the quart and a
half of water. Give this gently at first, but
eventually--that is, after the period when
there has been the ability for a movement--use
the colon tube. Then we would take internally
--after the Oil Packs and the enema--a tablespoonful of Olive Oil." 1523-9

"Consider that which takes place from the use
of the oil pack and its influence upon the
body, and something of the emotion experienced
may be partially understood.
"Oil is that which constitutes, in a form, the
nature of activity between the functionings
of the organs of the system as related to
activity. Much in the same manner as oil would
act upon an inanimate object--it acts as a
limbering agent, allowing movement, motion,
which may be had by inanimate machinery motion.
This is the same effect had upon that which
is now animated by spirit. This movement, then,
was the reflection of the abilities of the
spirit of ANIMATE activity as is controlled
through the emotions of mind, or the activity
of mind between spirit and matter." 1523-15

To understand how and why castor oil stimulates
normal peristalsis, let us examine the causes for the
suspension of peristalsis. Nature intended the bulk
in the foods we eat to stimulate the muscles of the
intestines to do their work. Today's modern diet of
highly refined foods, designed for easier assimilation,

has robbed the contents of the intestines of the necessary bulk. Instead of working properly, these muscles become flaccid and lazy through the lack of exercise; they work less and less, slower and slower, until finally their effectiveness results in constipation, auto-intoxication, and all the other dreaded diseases which follow naturally when the system is weakened through constant absorption of the poisons formed in the colon.

Castor Oil Packs produces peristalsis because it supplies lubrication for activity of movement. When this lubrication from the Castor Oil Packs passes into the colon, the peristalsis muscles find that they are receiving a natural stimulation, and therefore, they get to work!

The result is a thorough, natural and complete movement of the bowels; the eliminations are easier, because they are perfectly natural, and because of the wonderful lubricating qualities of Castor Oil, the passage of the body's waste are smooth and effortless. Since the peristalsis muscles, like all the other muscles of the body, are benefited and strengthened by exercise, this restoration of normal peristalsis helps the colon regain its full power and health.

The test of natural bowel evacuation is in the character of the stool. A well-formed stool indicates that the action was in accordance with nature's dictates. A loosely formed stool indicates force and probable injury. Here is another nature-test by which you can determine the efficiency of bulk food. It not only produces regular elimination, but it also does it naturally!

First of all--and this may be a shock to a great many of you--one elimination a day is really not enough! (John Harvey Kellogg of Battle Creek is the authority of that statement.) If you eat three meals a day, it means that waste matter reaches your intestines three times a day; the poisonous waste from two of your meals lingers in the body too long. It would be better for your well-being if you had two or three complete and thorough evacuations each day--if your body eliminated its waste as soon as it accumulated. Here is why.

The intestines are not only the sewerage system of the body, but they are also the feeding grounds of the blood! Innumerable tiny blood vessels feed from the nourishing elements of the foods we eat--from the very spot where these elements have been sorted from the waste matter which this food contained. As long as waste matter is eliminated promptly and the intestines kept clean, the blood absorbs only nourishment. Let us see what happens when waste matter is allowed to accumulate.

You have observed what happens to foods when it is kept too long in a warm place--it spoils, turns putrid and rots, and becomes unfit to eat. Practically the same process goes on when the waste accumulates in your intestines. Swiftly, due to the body's heat, this waste decomposes, rotting and putrefying ever so much more rapidly than it would outside of the body; the waste matter throws off acute toxic poisons which, in large quantities are actually deadly! The blood, led to the intestines to take on nourishment, is also loaded down with these poisons and carries them widespread throughout the body. Headaches, dullness, and autointixication are the immediate results; but that is only half the danger. It is the function of the blood not only to rebuild and to nourish every organ of the body, it must also fight the germs of disease.

Weakened by the ever constant battle against the poisons absorbed from the intestinal tract, the blood is unable to defeat the disease germs which it must also fight. You become the easy victim of one of the many malignant diseases which, if you were in really good health, your blood would have no difficulty for overcoming such parasites.

Can you realize the far-reaching effects of such apparently unimportant and common ailment as constipation; the tremendous importance of the complete and thorough internal cleanliness as obtained through the process of proper elimination.

"Q.- Should anything be taken for elimination?
"A.- Correct your eliminations better by diet
than by taking eliminants, when possible. If

If not possible to correct otherwise, take an eliminant, but alter between one time a vegetable laxative and the next time a mineral eliminant. But these elimination problems will be bettered if a great deal of the raw vegetables are used and not so much of meats; but do eat fish, fowl, and lamb occasionally... don't fry it." 3381-1

"A vegetable as well as a mineral laxative should be alternated in the use of alkalizers, or the agents taken for increasing eliminations through the alimentary canal. It is well for those requiring any laxative to change about. Have a mineral and again the vegetable compound, so there is the better balance kept, and neither become so necessary or more serious, will not destroy entirely the sphincter activities of the muscular forces of the alimentary canal." 849-67

"Rather than so much Castoria (vegetable base) in the present--for this can be irritating, of course--we would occasionally change to other eliminants. As we have indicated for other bodies, it is well to alternate these rather than continuing to take just one type of eliminant. Occasionally, then, we would take the Milk of Bismuth, a teaspoonful with a few drops of Elixir of Lacerated Pepsin in same, stirred in half a glass of water. This is to cleanse the system, or to absorb the poisons. Then afterward it would be necessary to take small doses of Eno Salts or Sal Hepatica. The Sal Hepatica of course is partially mineral, while the Eno Salts is practically all vegetable, or fruit salts, see?" 264-48

Therefore:

"Set up better eliminations by the use of those foods that tend to produce better drainages

...*laxative foods such as a great deal of pieplant whenever obtainable, raisins, stewed and prepared in other foods, a great deal of the black figs and the white and purple also, and the prunes and prune preparation.*"

3336-1

Again: (we repeat)

"...*for would the assimilations and the eliminations be kept nearer to normal in the human family, the days of life might be extended to whatever period desired; for the system is builded by the assimilations of that which it takes within--and it is able to bring resuscitation so long as the eliminations do not hinder.*" 311-4

"*For as indicated ever, there is gradually a replenishing of every portion of the body, if the proper balance is kept in the system so that the eliminations and assimilations are such that each portion of the system may reproduce itself.*" 4061-1

"*Know that even at this period in the experience of the body there is that within the body which WILL replenish, if the body is kept cleansed from the impurities of poor eliminations.*" 1464-1

"*Hence we would continue the care as to activities related to the diet, as related to associations with others, as related to the abuses of influences in filling the system with destructive forces; and we will find we will keep this body a continuity not only of the re-creative force within self but of the vital active forces in same.*" 1554-4

Constipation is characterized by sluggish action of the bowels. For some reason the evacuation of waste matter from the large intestines has become difficult.

Normally an individual should have a copious movement of the bowels twice in twenty-four hours--3 times is much better, or after every meal.

Constipation has become so common among people of civilized countries that this has been called "the age of constipation." At least three-quarters of the chronic patients requesting readings from Cayce, ailed from chronic constipation in its worst forms. Many of them tell that they have not had a natural movement of the bowels for many years. This alone is sufficient to show that the ordinary methods of living and of treating human ills are faulty and inadequate to say the least.

While itself only a symptom of failure on the part of the muscles of the large intestines, constipation becomes in turn one of the primary causes of other constitutional diseases. The inactivity of the eliminating organs, the skin, the kidneys and bowels causes the retention of waste and morbid matter which results in body poisoning, and auto-intoxication. The system of treatment which cannot restore the normal activity of the organs of cleansing cannot accomplish anything else.

The medical treatment of constipation, consists largely in the administering of laxatives and cathartics, gives only temporary relief and tends to benumb and paralyze the intestines much more completely. So all laxatives and purgatives are poisonous and destructive to the system, or they would not produce any peculiar drastic effects. They do not act upon the system but the system reacts from the drugs. Being poisons, the body tries to expel these enemies to health and life by copiuous excretions from the liver and from the walls of the intestines. This eventually produces an evacuation of the contents of the bowels, but every time such violent artificial stimulation is restored, the liver, the membraneous linings of the intestinal tract and the nerves which supply them, become more benumbed and more inactive. Many cases of inflammation of the intestines--colitis, and others-- are simply due to inflammation injuries, due to the use of drastic drugs.

The inflammation of the tender linings of the intestines is only one of the evils. The violent and drastic stimulation following drugging causes those muscles of the digestive system to shrink, shrivel up, and become flabby

This is found most frequently in people who have habitually utilized drugs having a very paralyzing effect upon the digestive tract. The acute catarrhal conditions characterized by the frequent purging are indicated by recurring attacks of diarrhea and mucous passing in the stools, etc.

Mental and emotional conditions exert a powerful influence upon the alimentary tract. Certain emotions have a benumbing, others a stimulating effect upon the secretions and the peristaltic action of the bowels. A few days ago I read about certain experiments made with living animals. X-rays pictures were taken of a healthy cat whose peristaltic movements were normally active. The animal was suddenly confronted with an angry dog barking at her fiercely. Instantly, as the hairs on her body went up as a result of sudden fright and anger, the peristaltic action of the stomach and bowels ceased entirely and did not revive until the animal had thoroughly recovered from its emotional excitement. It also has been proved by experiments on living animals that sudden emotional excitement stops the secretion of gastric and pancreatic juices.

It must be understood that the first requisite in the treatment of any disorder, and especially of constipation, is a change in not only the diet but also a change in our attitudes and emotions.

Therefore, we should resort to colon flushing only as a crutch in the beginning of treatment until the intestines become alive and active under natural diet and treatment. It is then advisable to resort to flushing only when necessary since it is not curative in any way whatsoever.

OSTEOPATHY

Osteopathy is one of the most important branches of natural healing. By itself, however, it is not all-sufficient because it deals only with the mechanical treatment of disease, and not with the chemical and thermal, nor with the mental and psychical.

The best osteopathic treatment cannot make good for the bad effects of an unbalanced diet, which contains an excessive amount of the poison-producing materials, and which is deficient in the all-important positive mineral elements or "organic salts." Just as surely as mental therapeutics and a pure natural diet cannot set dislocated bones and joints, and just as surely as it is impossible to cure monomania and obsession, or to supply iron, potash and sodium to the blood, by correcting spinal lesions only.

The trouble with many osteopathic schools and their graduates is that they adhere too closely to the mechanical theory and treatment of disease; that they reject practically all natural methods of treatment aside from manipulation, and that their practitioners, since they find manipulation by itself insufficient in many cases, show a strong tendency to fall back upon the old-school methods of drugging and surgical treatments.

In order to do justice to our readers and not neglect our responsibilities towards them, we must state that in the treatment of disease all that is good should be utilized in all of the various methods for promoting natural healing. In serious chronic cases any single one of these methods--whether it be pure-food diet, hydrotherapy, massage, osteopathy, mental therapeutics or homeopathy--is not sufficient by itself to achieve perfect results, or to rather produce them quickly enough. To use an illustration:

Suppose a wagon full of merchandise requires the combined strength of 7 horses to move it, and suppose that number of horses are available, would it not be foolish to try and move the load with one or three or even five horses? Would not common sense dictate that to save time and effort we must put all 7 horses to at once in the initial try.

In the natural healing procedures, every one of the different natural methods of treatment is complemented and assisted by all of the others, as exemplified in the case histories of the Cayce readings.

For instance, case history of # 1123-2 as given on February 1, 1937, follows in its entirety.

"Mr. Cayce: Yes--we have the body, (1123).

"Now, as we find, there are very definite disturbances in the physical forces of this body,

"As we find, these have arisen from properties injected for preventions in the physical reactions of the body. Hence those portions of the body have become involved from which assimilations produce those elements necessary for the replenishing of organs, of activity, of all forces of the body.

"So the whole of the left portion of the body is involved, but affectation arises from the right portion--or caecum area.

"Not the affectation of the vermiform appendage but rather that from which such conditions may arise eventually, without correction; yet involving more the lacteal area and the gall duct and the glandular system.

"From same then very poor digestion arises at times, also a low blood pressure, a very slow pulsation and a general anemia.

"These as we find are those disturbing forces in this body.

"As we find then, in making applications those things that may be helpful, we must take into consideration portions of the system involved and build to that as will stimulate the activity for a more perfect balance; and allow the system through its coordination to adjust the conditions.

"Hence from the osteopathic standpoint, first corrections must be made in the coccyx area, in the 4th lumbar; and then in the 1st, 2nd and 3rd dorsal area. At the same time, or during these periods (we wouldn't give these

*closer together than twice a week), or just
before these corrections are made, we would
apply Castor Oil Packs over the caecum and the
liver area, for half an hour, just as hot as
the body can stand, see?*

*"After these are applied (let the body rest
for a period, twenty to thirty minutes), then
make the adjustments; and we will find it will
make a great deal of difference in the manner
in which there are the reactions to the eliminations and assimilations of the system.*

*"Take internally the Ventriculin with Iron.
This we would take three times each week, not
a heaping teaspoonful but rather a level teaspoonful. This is to add to the elements of the
body the ability for those activities upon the
organs of the system to produce for the blood
supply a better stamina, more of that hormone
within the blood that strengthens the vitality
of the whole of the assimilating system.*

*"These we would keep up (that is, the manipu-
lations, the oil packs, also the taking of the
Ventriculin to raise the blood pressure, to
increase the blood supply, and then repeat the
whole course.*

*"And we would find that these create, with the
keeping of alkalinity, those abilities for the
body to resist cold.*

*"Do not give (as there is at times indicated
in the body's system) citrus fruit juices and
cereals at the same meal, or even the same
day--for this body! But a portion of the week
have citrus fruit juices as the basis of the
morning meal, or during the day, and the other
portion of the week have the crushed wheat or
cracked wheat (but well cooked) as the basis
of the morning meal--never the two together.*

*"Let one meal each day, or the greater portion
of it, consists of raw vegetables. Celery,
lettuce, tomatoes, radish, onions--any or all
of these should be the greater part of the
whole meal each day at least.*

*"Do these and as we find we will soon see a
much bettered condition for this body, (1123).
"We are through for the present." 1123-2*

One of the primary objects of osteopathy is to
correct bony lesions. If any one of the bones in the
body is out of place, it presses or "impinges" upon
neighboring structures and tissues and obstruct blood,
nerve, and lymphatic vessels, thus interfering with
the functions of cells and organs and inhibiting the
natural flow of the vital fluids and nerve currents.

The harmful results of displacements or deviations
from the normal are of especial importance when the
spinal column is affected.

This structure is made up of thirty-three separate
bones, more or less loosely jointed together by means
of cartilaginous substance in such a way that they
form a hollow tube which contains the spinal cord.

After the nerve trunks, branching out from the
spinal cord, pass through these openings, they divide
and subdivide into millions of branches, fibers, and
filaments, which carry vital energy and nerve impulses
to and from every cell in the human body.

If, therefore, any of the vertebrae of the spinal
column became dislocated or "luxated," an abnormal
pressure will be exerted upon the nerve trunks and
blood vessels passing between them to and from the
spinal cord.

In accordance with certain physiological laws,
irritation at any point along the course of a nerve is
communicated to all the branches of that nerve similar
to the way an electric current, applied at any point of
a network of copper wires, if not checked or diverted,
will travel over all wires connected with that part.

Thus abnormal pressure upon and the consequent
irritation of a nerve trunk will be transmitted to all
the branches of that nerve and carried to all the cells
and organs supplied by that particular nerve trunk
and its branches, resulting in inflammation, pain, and
abnormal function in the different parts.

In accordance with the same physiological law,
if a nerve is benumbed and paralyzed at any point along

its course, the nerve and its branches beyond this point of interference and all the structures depending upon them for their supply of nerve force will also be numbed and paralyzed.

The pressure of luxated bones on nerves or blood vessels may be illustrated by the effect of compression upon a rubber hose through which water is flowing. Stepping upon the hose will stop the flow of water; in like manner abnormal pressure or impingement upon nerves or blood and lymph vessels interfere with the flow of vital currents. Thus the tissues and organs depending upon these currents for their blood and nerve supply are deprived of sufficient nourishment, proper drainage, and of the communication with headquarters in the brain and with the spinal cord.

There can be but one remedy for such mechanical interference, and that consists in replacing or adjusting the dislocated bones where they belong through treatment by a trained osteopath.

"Let's describe this for a second, that the entity or body here may understand, as well as the one making the stimulation.

"Along the cerebro-spinal system we find segments. These are cushioned. Not that the segment itself is awry, but through each segment there arise an impulse or a nerve connection between it and the sympathetic system—or the nerves running parallel with same. Through the sympathetic system (as it is called, or those centers not encased in cerebro-spinal system) are the connections with the cerebro-spinal system.

"Then, in each center—that is, of the segment where these connect—there are tiny bursa, or a plasm of nerve reaction. This becomes congested, or slow in its activity to each portion of the system. For, each organ, each gland of the system, receives impulses through this manner for its activity.

"Hence we find there are reactions to every portion of the system by suggestion, mentally,

and by the environment and surroundings.

"Also we find that a reaction may be stimulated INTERNALLY to the organs of the body, by injection of properties or foods, or by the activities of same.

"We also find the reflex from these internally to the brain centers.

"Then the SCIENCE of osteopathy is not merely the punching in a certain segment, or the cracking of the bones, but it is the keeping of a BALANCE--by the touch--between the sympathetic and the cerebro-spinal system! THAT is real osteopathy.

"With the adjustments made in this way and manner, we will find not only helpful influences but healing and an aid to any condition that may exist in the body--unless there is a broken bone or the like!" 1158-24

"For the moment, let's understand what the sympathetic and the cerebro-spinal nervous system are within the human body.

"In the cerebro-spinal centers, here we have the brain, the spinal cord--which enters through all the cerebro-spinal system, passing through each vertebra, and the impingement on same often cause much of the distress to the body-physical. This may be presented as the physical organism.

"There is lying along each side of the cerebro-spinal system a series, or on either side a cord known as the sympathetic nervous system. Not within the structural portions, but connecting with same at definite points; though in many points connecting with same but at definite points.

"The activities of these:

"The cerebro-spinal, the nerve cord itself, acts for the physical attributes of the body through the impulses.

"The sympathetic is the greater impulsive system.

"Each segment connects with a centralized area between the sympathetic and the cerebrospinal systems, or in the spinal cord impulse itself. In specific centers there runs a connecting link between the segments. And such an one exists in this particular center as we have indicated (2nd and 3rd dorsal).

"In each of those areas called a ganglion there is a bursa, or a small portion of nerves tissue that acts as a regulator or a conductor, or as a director of impulses from the nerve forces to the organs of the body that are affected by this portion of the nervous system.

"Not that any one organ, any one functioning of an organ, receives all its impulse from one ganglion or one center along the spine; but that these slowing up by a deficiency in the activity because of pressure produce--as here--a lesion, or an attempt of the blood flow (that is, the lymph and emunctory flow) to shield any injured portion of any pressure. This ofttimes increases the amount of pressure to other portions of the body." 1120-2

Therefore:

"...nearly all derangements, save mental forces, come from some center being so separated by pressure that another functioning position in body becomes either deranged by lack of nutriment received or by over stimulus and producing too much of another character..."
1447-1

"Now the abnormal conditions as we find in this body have to do with the nervous systems and the effect as produced in the body by those conditions, both to the brain itself in its functioning and to some portions of the system as traversed by the nerves governing those conditions." 151-1

"Q.- What causes the dizziness, and why the headaches continue?

"A.-The inability of coordination between the sympathetic and cerebro-spinal as related to those of the sensory system." 153-2

"You tie up nerves along the spine what do you usually find, in any electrical charge? Corrosion as will appear side of a connection--and it may appear in thine own body. For the nerves are the electrical system of the body. Hence this discharge is from the lack of poisons being carried through their proper channels."
3641-1

Then:

"...when we have hindrances, as is designated or seen here with this body, where nerves fail to receive proper incentives, the reaction from those organs or those portions of the system supplied by that nerve energy suffers in its cycle of functioning." 108-2

"...the strain between the physical and mental, with the spiritual attributes of the individual, finds expression not only in the brain itself, but in that of the sympathetic system or the brain manifestation of soul forces in the body." 4566-1

Once again:

"There is no form of physical mechano-therapy so near in accord with NATURE'S measures as the correctly given osteopathic adjustments. Others may say what they may, but prove it by watching those who have them regularly and depend upon them!" 1158-31

Therefore, by means of osteopathy we are enabled to stimulate, relax, or inhibit nerves and nerve centers, and through these the cells and organs which they supply in any part of the body. This is accomplished by certain manipulations applied to the nerves and nerve centers along the spine, where they come nearest to the surface and can be influenced by manipulative treatment.

> *"For as understood by the body, and by the one that would make the mechanical or osteopathic adjustments, or the massage or masseuse activity, there is every force in the body to recreate its own self--if the various portions of the system are coordinating and cooperating one with another.*
>
> *"Hence the reason why, as we have so oft given from the sources here, the mechanical adjustments as may be administered by a thorough or serious osteopathic manipulator may nearer adjust the system for its perfect unison of activity than most any other means--save under acute or specific conditions; and even then the more oft such become necessary.*
>
> *"...we will find the system is enabled, through these activities (osteopathic manipulation)-- by the proper diet--to assimilate and replenish all those forces that may be supplied through chemical or drug activities.*
>
> *"...then the mechanical applications for this body would be more in order than taking other conditions (drugs) in same." 1158-11*

In accordance with the before mentioned law, stimulation applied to the nerves and nerve centers in close proximity to the spinal column, are carried over all the branches and filaments of these nerves into the innermost recesses of the body, thus stimulating and invigorating the internal cells and organs to intensified and more normal activity.

Similarly, the relaxing or inhibitory treatment applied to the nerve centers along the spinal column is communicated to the cells and organs in the interior of the body, thus soothing and relieving pain, hyperactivity, and congestion in the parts affected by inflammatory and feverish processes.

The character of the osteopathic treatments are similarly outlined in the Cayce readings.

"*The osteopathic treatments are of these characters:*
(1)   "*There are those where stimulation of ganglia as related to the functioning of organs will assist in increasing the circulation to produce drainage.*
(2)   "*Or there may be such as to PREVENT drainage, or to prevent activity in this direction.*
(3)   "*And there are those where specific mechanical adjustments may be made.*" 849-22

Examples of the above treatments follow:

(1)   "*We would have treatments by massage, or of the chiropractic or osteopathic nature, or a combination of these, to set up drainages in the system; particularly as related to better activity of the liver and the gall duct, and as the general eliminating system.*
Take these at least twice or three times a week for at least fifteen such treatments or adjustments; then leave off for a period of two weeks; and then take another course of an equal period of time." 2383-2

(2)   "*Each week have a thorough relaxing treatment osteopathically. This should never be a stimulating treatment, and should not be done so as to get through with it in two or three minutes; but slowly, easily, relax the body, first, in the 1st, 2nd, 3rd, 4th cervicals-- on either side of same; then the 1st, 2nd, 3rd, 4th dorsals--then in the 9th dorsal. These should be released, but relaxed and then the releasing. This should require at least twenty to thirty minutes for a gentle massage to relax the body thoroughly.*" 3386-1

(3)   "*The osteopath may give the adjustments provided the anatomy of conditions is understood by such an operator. First we would give, X-ray the condition of the cerebro-spinal system, especially in the region of the 6th,*

*7th, 8th, 9th, 10th and 11th dorsal. The 9th
will be the segment found upon which first
adjustments should be made. Rather than of
massage, adjust, that the impingement as is
caused by the position of segment may be
relieved.*

*"The properties as are being at present
accorded the system, keep these until the
system shows response to these properties as
outlined. Then, gradually diminish, diminishing the injections for the capillary circulation first, but gradually diminishing all.
This, we will find, will give the correct
assimilation and assists the eliminations to
become normal."* 4156-2

Therefore:

*"...the one who gives the osteopathic treat-
ments, if thoroughly acquainted with his
business (though many think they are when they
are not) will find that there are centers or
areas from which both the cerebro-spinal and
the sympathetic or vegetative nerve system
form conjunctions. If specific treatments are
given and there is not a coordination of those
plexus or areas where the specific conjunctions
are made, these may tend to contract the body
rather than relax same. Hence there should be
the consideration of all of these when treatments are given."* 2094-2

It is certainly true that the misapplication of
treatment as well as the displacement of the spinal
vertabrae and the resulting impingement on nerves and
blood vessels may help bring about acute inflammatory
processes; but it is also true that the latter through
the irritations of muscles and ligaments attached to
the spinal vertebrae, may pull these bones out of
their proper alignment. In such cases the vertebrae
reassume their natural position after the inflammatory
processes (and there with the tension on the spinal

muscles) had subsided. If this readjustment does not take place spontaneously, it must then, of course, be brought about by manipulative treatment.

A similar phenomena of displacement and readjustment may be observed in the iris of the eye. Just before the development and during the course of an acute disease in any part or organ of the body, the corresponding area in the iris becomes clouded with white lines and flakes. The inflammatory processes going on in the body are reproduced in the eye. The congestion in the lower layers of the iris presses the nerve fibers of the upper layer above the surface level. These protuding fibers have a white appearance and produce the white signs of acute diseases and healing crises.

When the inflammatory processes in the body and the corresponding congestion in the iris subside, the nerve fibers sink back into their normal position, the white signs of inflammation disappear, and the surface of the iris presents once more its usual blue or brown appearance.

In similar manner the vertabrae of the spine do reassume their normal position after all the tension exerted upon them by the inflammatory processes has subsided.

We do not wish to convey the impression that manipulation, properly applied, may not be very helpful in the treatment of acute diseases. But we must persist in claiming that the inflammatory processes, after they have once started, must not be checked or suppressed, and that the most essential part of natural treatment consists in fasting, massage and hydrotherapy applications, because all these promote the elimination of morbid matter more thouroughly than any other method of treatment.

The underlying causes of disease must be removed before a normal condition can be brought about. Suppose then, the chiropracter or osteopath should succeed in stopping a fever instantly. The patient would still continue to "load up" more morbid materials, and it would only be a matter of time until the morbid accumulations in the body would excite new acute reactions,

necessitating more adjustments. This may be fine for
the practitioner, but what about the patient? In the
long run it can have only one result, and it is that
known as chronic disease.

"Clear the body as you do the mind of those
things that have hindered...physically are the
poor eliminations. Set up better eliminations
in this body. This is why osteopathy and hydrotherapy come nearer to being the basis of all
needed treatments for physical disabilities."
                                            2854-5

"Q.- Should the adjustments be made osteopatically?
"A.- Osteopatically, of course; for this is the
method by which coordination is made between
various centers along the system. This is the
variation between the different schools in
adjustment or massage. Some schools of adjustment work on the theory that if you relieve
the pressure in one area the other naturally
adjusts itself! But the osteopathic method
makes the coordination. Then, we find the
osteopathic and the neuropathic being the
greater beneficial applications in such fields
of activity." 683-2

"Q.- How often should the osteopathic treatment be given?
"A.- This will depend upon the needs of the
body. As we find, the better manner is to have
treatments for two or three weeks, then a rest
period for a week or two weeks, and then begin
the treatments again--these at least twice a
week. This adds to the body, allowing the
adjustments. For manipulative forces osteopa-
cally given, unless there is necessity for
corrections, only assist the body in breaking
up congestion or congested areas or in assist-
ing ganglia under stress or strain to be so
adjusted that the elimination or drainages in
portions of the body are set up and stimulation

to *active functioning organs is produced.
These have been given properly. If the body
will adhere to these suggestions in a consistent manner, we will find relief in same."*
                                    1110-4
Therefore:

*"Once a week or twice a week for two or three
weeks, leave off for a period of a month to
six weeks and then have again. Such a manner
as we find is better, especially for the adult
or the older patient."* 1158-11

*"As indicated. For this body, these are best
taken in series. When they are taken, for the
month that they would be taken, take six. Then
it may be two months before they may again be
necessary."* 1158-31

CHIROPRACTIC

Chiropractic, an offspring of osteopathy, endeavors to accomplish the correction of spinal lesions by sudden, powerful "thrust" on the dislocated bones; but this treatment has to be applied very carefully lest it becomes exceedingly painful, and quite dangerous.

Such forceful manipulation may be indicated where the dislocation of vertebrae is due to an accident or an act of violence or of forceful play. Then another act of violence or force may be sufficient to correct the spinal lesion, replace the vertebrae in its normal position, and thus relieve the pressure upon blood vessels and nerves.

But where spinal lesions have been in existence for long periods of time, the muscles and ligaments attached to the vertebrae have become contracted and shortened on the one side, and abnormally relaxed and lengthened on the other side.

If in such cases the bones are thrust into place by main force, the contracted muscles and ligaments will soon pull them out of place again.

Furthermore, the forcible adjustment of bones which have been out of place for a long time and which are held in their abnormal positions by newly-formed connective tissue, often causes great pain and can be actually dangerous and injurious on account of the resistance offered by the newly-formed tissues. They may be lacerated by such violent manipulation, also.

What has just been said is true of osteopathic as well as chiropractic treatment. Here also violent manipulation and adjustment may prove unnecessarily painful and followed by injurious side-effects.

The more gradual natural healing method of the combined massage and osteopathic treatment, is therefore, to be preferred, as it softens and relaxes the contracted muscles and ligaments, and gives the tissues new life and tonicity. When through the more general and massage-like manipulations, the muscles, fleshy tissues, and ligaments attached to the dislocated bones have become more normal, the vertebrae of other bony structures, after being put in place, will be more likely to remain in their normal alignment.

"In meeting the needs, then, we would find that--with the proper adjustments, either properly chiropractically made, or better with the proper manipulation and adjustment osteopathically made--the body would show material improvement, would there be the same precautions taken with the invigorating as will be felt from same, as there has been heretofore --with the diet, the activities, the exercises and the eliminations. These may be aided by addition of varied properties. This we would find, would aid materially." 5420-1

"Occasionally we would have corrections in a chiropractic manner, and especially as to the pressures about the lower lumbar and the coccyx area; coordinating these with the area in the cervicals where the cardiac and the sympathetic forces cross to the head and nerve forces of the body. These we would take for one to two weeks, then we would rest or leave off for a like period, you see, and then begin again." 840-1

"After removing the Pack, sponge off the area with a rather strong soda water. Then massage the same area gently, by a masseuse or an osteopath or one well-trained in physiotherapy or neuropathic massage. Little should be applied to the spine in the beginning, but be careful that the connections from the sixth dorsal to the first cervical are in alignment. Test these by the radioclast, or the instrument usually used by the chiropractic profession to indicate position of segments. This is a very good instrument and should be used more often by other professions also that make mechanical adjustments." 3210-1

In justice to chiropractic it must be said that the more adcanced chiropractic schools, such as the Universal Chiropractic College in Davenpot, Io., have learned this lesson and have greatly modified the harsh treatment as taught and practiced by the originators of this system. They also teach along with the purely manipulative treatment the principles of other natural methods of healing.

While considering the theory and practical application of manipulative treatment, it must not ever be overlooked that natural living tends of itself to make the human body normal in structure and functions.

When through a natural diet the blood has become purified and more normal in its constituents, and when by means of hydrotherapy, air and sun baths, physical exercise, etc., the organism in general thus becomes invigorated and regenerated. The many lesions in the bony structure have adjusted themselves, exactly as the signs of disease conditions have completly disappeared from the body

This is especially true of the bodies of the very young, whose bony structures are still plastic-like and in the process of development. In a number of instances crooked and deformed limbs and spines have straighten out under the beneficial influence of the natural regime even without special manipulative treatment.

In a manner the vertabrae of the spine reassume their normal position after the tension exerted upon them by the inflammatory process has subsided.

Therefore, the underlying causes of disease must be removed before we can bring about a normal condition of the organism.

"For this particular body we recommend that treatment be continued by the present Chiropractor. We would ordinarily suggest osteopathy, but there are chiropractors and chiropractors. This one is very good; don't lose him, he understands this body." 5211-1

HOMEOPATHY

True homeopathic medicines in high-potency doses are so highly refined and rarefied that they cannot possible produce harmful effects or suppress nature's cleansing and healing efforts; on the contrary, if employed according to the law of homeopathy: "Like Cures Like," they assist in producing acute reactions or "healing crises," thus aiding nature in the work of purification and repair of the body.

Homeopathy works with the laws of healing, not against them. "Similia similibus curantur" ("like cures like") translated into practice means that a drug capable of producing a certain set of disease symptoms in a healthy body, when given in large, physiological doses, will relieve or cure a similar set of symptoms in the disease organism if the drug is given in small, homeopathic doses.

For instance, belladonna, given in large, poisonous doses to a healthy person, will cause a peculiar headache with sharp, stabbing pains in forehead and temples, high fever, violent delirium, dilation of the pupils, dryness and rawness of the throat, scarlet redness of the skin, and extreme sensitiveness to the light, sudden jars and noises.

It will be observed that this is a fair picture of a typical case of scarlet fever patient exhibiting in a marked degree three or more of the above described symptoms: would give a trituration of belladonna, say 6X. In numberless cases the fever has subsided and its symptoms have rapidly disappeared under such treatment.

The reader may say: "I do not see any difference between this and the allopathic suppression of disease by drugs."

There is a great big difference. The allopathic physician may use the same remedy, belladonna, in the same case, but he will give from ten to twenty drops of tincture of belladonna, repeated every three or four hours. These doses are from twenty to forty thousand times stronger than the homeopathic 3X or 6X.

Herein lies the difference. The allopathic dose

allays the fever symptoms by paralyzing the organism as a whole and the different vital organs, and their functions in particular. This is frequently admitted in every allopathic materia medica. But by such dosing nature is forcibly interrupted in her valid efforts of cleansing and healing; the acute reaction is suppressed but not in any way cured.

If fever is a healing effort of nature, it may be controlled and modified, but must not be suppressed. A minute dose of homeopathic belladonna, acting on the innermost cells of the organism, which the coarser allopathic doses would paralyze, will stimulate these cells to effort in the right direction. It so brings about conditions similar to those produced by nature, and thus assists her; this is cooperation instead of counter-operation.

After this brief discussion of the practical application of homeopathy, let us now ascertain as to how far its laws and theories agree with and corroborate the laws and principles of the natural healing, natural application philosophy.

Hahnemann discovered the law of "like cures like" accidently, while investigating the effects of quinine on the human organism. Ever since then it has been applied successfully by him and his followers in the treatment of human ailments.

However, this law has been used empirically. Neither in the "Organon" nor in any other writings or teachings of Hahnemann and the homeopathic school can be found a clear and concise explanation of why "like cures like." The proof offered has been negative rather than positive.

With the aid of the three laws of cure, we shall endeavor to give the reasons and furnish the proofs for the matter in question. The laws alluded to are: The Law of Cure; The Law of Dual Effect; and The Law of Crises.

"Like cures like" is only another way of stating the fundamental law of natural healing: "Every acute disease is the result of a cleansing and an healing effort of nature."

If a certain set of disease symptoms are the

result of a healing effort of nature, and if given a remedy which produces the same or similar symptoms in the system, is it not aiding nature in her attempt to overcome the abnormal conditions?

In such a case, the indicated homeopathic remedy will not suppress the acute reaction, but it will help it along, thus accelerating and hastening the curative process of healing and cure.

In the last analysis, disease resides in the cell. The well-being of the organism as a whole is dependent upon the health of the individual cells of which it is composed.

In order to cure the man, we must free the cell of its encumbrances. Elimination must begin in the cell, not in the organs of depuration. Laxatives and cathartics, by irritating the digestive tract, may cause a forced evacuation of the contents of the intestinal canal, but they do not eliminate the poisons which clog cells and tissues.

In stubborn chronic diseases, when the cells are too weak to throw off the latent encumbrances of their own accord, a well chosen homeopathic remedy is often of great service in arousing them to acute reaction.

The question now arises: How large or how small must be the dose in order to affect the minute cells?

In the administration of medicines, the size of the dose is adjusted to the size of the patient. If half a grain of a certain drug is the normal dose for an adult, the proper dose of the same drug for a small infant, say, less than a year old, may be about one twenty-fifth part of the adult dose. How small, in proportion, should then be the dose given to a cell a billion times as small as the infant baby.

But this is how allopathy effects its fictitious cures. It suppresses inflammatory processes by paralyzing the cells and organs and their activities.

Homeopathy adapts the smallness of the dose to the smallness of the cell which is to be treated. Herein lies the reasonableness of high potency doses.

The cell resembles man not only in physical and physiological aspects, but also in regard to the whole law, that is, the physical, mental, spiritual law.

"Just as the impressions to the whole of the organism, for each cell of the blood stream, each corpuscle, is a whole universe in itself."
                                        341-31
"For each cell in the atomic force of the body is as a world of its own, and each one--each cell--being in perfect unison, may build to that (which is) necessary to reconstruct the forces of the body in all its needs...."93-1

"Remember, every cell of the body is a universe in itself, with all the elements necessary for the creating of, the bringing into being that necessary. For is not the human body the effect of all creation?" 1158-22

"He (entity) finds himself, then a counterpart, a shadow of all that is; and that within his own self. EACH CELL of its body is but a miniature of the universe without its own body, its own cell of positive and negative force that applies to the material, the mental and the spiritual." 1776-1

Therefore:

"For as each cell in each atom of the body knows its purpose, if it is imbued with the spirit of LIFE, yet knoweth naught if it is condemned by the desires of the flesh only to its mere rote of activity--yet quickened by the Spirit bringeth, even as in thine experience, that of the unnatural to the natural."
                                        1158-5

Elimination, therefore, must commence in the cell and by virtue of the cell's personal effort. Its work cannot be done vicariously by drugs or the knife. Large, allopathic doses of medicine may be given with the idea of doing the work for the cell by violently stimulating or else paralyzing the organism as a whole or certain ones of the vital organs; but this is demoralizing and destructive to the cell. Those powerful doses calculated to affect the body and its organs as a whole make superfluous or paralyzes the individual efforts of the cells and tissues.

Alms-giving, prison sentences, and capital punishment have a similar allopathic effect on man, the individual cell of the social body. Instead of providing for him the proper environment and the opportunity for natural development and for working out his own salvation, they take this opportunity away from him and so weaken his personal effort making it quite impossible for him to make any progess.

Every agent affecting the human organism has two effects; a first, apparent, temporary one and a second lasting one. The second effect is directly opposite to the first.

Allopathy, in giving large, physiological doses, takes into consideration only the first, apparent effect of the drug, and thereby accomplishes long run results directly opposite to those which it desires to bring about. It produces the very conditions which it tries to cure. As an example, note the permanent effects of laxatives, stimulants, and sedatives upon the system.

On the other hand, the homeopathic physician may use the same remedies as the allopath, provided they produce symptoms similar to those of the disease. But he administers the different drugs in such minute doses that their first effect is noticed only as a slight homeopathic aggravation, while their second, lasting effect is relied upon to relieve and cure the disease.

In other words, homeopathy produces as the first effect, the condition like the disease, and counts on the second and lasting effect of the drug to bring about a permanent change.

If, in accordance with the law of dual effect as applied to drugs, the primary, temporary effect of the homeopathic remedy is equal to the disease, it is self-evident that the secondary, lasting effect of the remedy must be equal to the cure.

This law has been proven by homeopathy for over a hundred years. An experienced homeopathic prescriber would no more doubt it than he would doubt the law of gravitation.

Therefore, if the remedy is well chosen in accord with the law of "like cures like," the first homeopathic aggravation, which corresponds to the crisis of natural healing, will be followed by a speedy and perfect readjustment. Nature has her way, the disorder runs its course, and the return to normal conditions will be quicker and more perfect than if the homeopathic remedy had not been employed or if nature's healing processes had been forcibly interrupted and suppressed by large and poisonous allopathic doses. Homeopathy assists nature by the removing of old encumbrances, whereas allopathy changes the acute and inflammatory healing effort into chronic destructive diseases.

"Q.- Would you consider the use of homeopathic remedies? Of compresses made from the juices of herbs? If so what would you suggest?
"A.- As we find, the use of these Oils AND the applications indicated for the allaying of the inflammatory forces as combined with same, would be the most effective in the special condition; see? 1623-4

"Hence, more often it will be found that the activity from what is known as the homeopathic doses is the better; even of allopathic medicine." 276-5

"Q.- Would it be advisable and useful if I prescribed and gave the "Homeopathic" remedies to my patients besides the regular treatment?
"A.- Remember what has just been given. If thoroughly understood, the Mechano-Therapy and Electro-Therapy should cover the broader field. To be sure, there are many instances where Homeopathy is indicated, we find that if this is to be used it will require more years in preparation." 3034-2

THE ECONOMICS OF HOMEOPATHY

The law of "like cures like" is of great practical importance from another point of view, namely, that of economics.

The best engineer is he who accomplishes the maximum of results with the minimum of explanation of force and with the least friction. The same is true of the physician and his remedies.

We have learned that drugs given in the coarse allopathic doses attack and affect the organism as a whole. If, for instance, there is a catarrhal affection of the serous and mucous membranes of the respiratory tract accompanied by fever, the allopath will give drugs in large doses to change this condition. He may accomplish his aim, but if so, he does it by paralyzing the heart, the respiratory centers, the red and white blood corpuscles, and the excreting cells of the mucous membranes. The body as a whole and certain parts in particular are saturated with the drug poison and are correspondingly weakened.

To state it another way: the large and allopathic dose paralyzes the whole organism in order to produce its fictitious cure. The small, homeopathic dose, on the other hand, goes right to the spot where it is needed, and by mild and harmless stimulation of the affected part, assists and supports the cells in their acute eliminative efforts.

Homeopathy medication, therefore, is not only curative in its effects, but also conservative and in the highest degree, economical.

Having proved the accuracy of Hahnemann's law of "like cures like," it would not be justifiable to omit homeopathy from the system of treatment for attaining natural healing. The attenuated homeopathic doses of certain drugs may be of great service in bringing about the acute reactions which are so earnestly desired, especially in the treatment of chronic diseases of long standing.

It is a known fact that in severe and obstinate conditions homeopathy is often apparently of no avail. But when the system has been purified and strengthened by natural methods, a rational vegetarian diet, hydrotherapy, osteopathy, massage, corrective exercise, air and sun baths, suggestive affirmations, and others, the homeopathic remedies will work with that much greater promptitude and effectiveness.

It is the combination of all the different healing factors which constitutes the perfect system of cure.

No disease condition, whether apparently hopeless or not, can ever be called incurable unless all these different healing factors, and properly combined and applied, have been given a thorough trial. It is no charlantanic boasting, but the simple truth, when we affirm that the different natural methods of treatment can and do cure so-called incurable diseases, providing that the patient possesses sufficient vitality as to react to the treatment and that the destruction of vital parts and organs has not advanced too far.

ELECTRO-THERAPY

There is an abundance of currently avaliable materials as well as research data regarding Electro-Therapy, but in this chapter, because of the limited space for such a wide subject area, it cannot in any way be fully covered. Therefore, we are limiting the coverage to the two electrical appliances described in the Edgar Cayce readings that we may have an idea of what this subject entails.

These appliances were mentioned in about ten percent of the physical readings, and are therefore an important adjunct in the treatment of disease and the healing process. There is a whole array of ailments for which the appliances were suggested, and at least 1000 references were made for their use in the Cayce readings.

The appliances are called the "wet cell battery" (formerly called the Wet Cell Appliance) and the "impedance device" (formerly called the Radio-Active Appliance). The wet cell battery was mentioned a few more times than the impedance device.

First a brief outline from the readings on the impedance device followed by an explanation of the wet cell battery.

> *"Mrs. C: You will have before you the reading (195-15) as given on (195), July 13, 1925, especially that portion of same in which there was given an appliance to be attached to this body each evening. You will please give us the specifics, in the benefitting of human ills to which the body is heir, for which this will be beneficial, and how this may be made and and distributed.*
> *"Mr. C: This, as we find, covers a great scope and field. In giving the conditions for which this would be a relief, we would first give that of the effect as is produced by such a combination unbalanced in the human organism, thus causing distress or disease to various portions of the body. The metal, as is seen,*

is the element as is understood, and known
already, to produce a form of electronic
vibrations, which to the body becomes a form
of motion for same, for we find (turning then
to the body) the human body is made up of
electronic vibrations, with each atom and
element of the body, each organ and organism
of same, having its electronic or unit vibration necessary for the sustenance of, and
equilibrium in, that particular organism. Each
unit, then, being a cell or a unit of life in
itself, with its capacity of reproducing
itself by the first form or law as is known
or reproduction, by division of same. When any
force in any organ, any element of the body,
becomes deficient in its ability to reproduce
that equilibrium necessary for the sustenance
of the physical existence and reproduction
of same, that portion becomes deficient,
deficient through electronic energy as is
necessary. This may become by injury, by disease, received from external forces; received
from internal forces by lack of eliminations
as are produced in the system, by the lack of
other agencies to meet the requirements of
same in the body.

"Now then, returning to the forces as are
applicable to the human ailments from such an
application of electronic forces as may be
received from a battery formation of carbon
steel, which becomes electronized by the ice
or cold, or water, partaking then of that
element, that vibration, in the Universal
elements of which man, human body, the greater
component forces make up of same.

"Iron--blood and the greater constituents of
force supplied from same. Cold, as from ice is
produced by the combination of other elements
necessary in the forces as is applied in man's
efforts in vibration to sustain human life.
The connection with same, then, produces that
equilibrium in the human body to relieve any

tension as is caused in the deficiency or over
proficiency of any electronic agent as is set
forth by any of the organisms as are found in
the human body. Then the action is as this:
An excess in one, by a unison of electronic
agencies, may be forced to assist that one
deficient. That one deficient may receive
sufficient of electronic agents, vibrations,
to the body to increase and assist the body
in gaining its perfect equilibrium. Acting as
the same principle to the body as this:
"The whole organism of the human body is made
up of such electronic forces as is necessary
for sufficient rest in that called sleep to
recuperate the energies of the whole body.
This application produces, then, that same
effect in the system.
"These specifies, then (for as we see would
cover many conditions as existing in system),
in this particular condition as expressed in
this as given for (195), we find is to reduce
the condition in strained centers wherein the
excess of vibration prevents the nominal or
normal vibration of the sensory or vibratory
system for the auditory forces of the body.
"Then for others, or for the general or specific conditions: Any catarrhal (and the body
is more heir to this than any other condition
existing in the forces of the human body)
condition existing in any portion of the
organism of the system, whether head, throat,
nasal, ear, lung, stomach, liver, kidneys or
unitary organs of the system. Any condition as
borders on any of these in which eliminations
produce a condition, this would be found
beneficial. Such as some of these: In the early
form of rheumatism, neuralgia, headaches, or
any condition produced by poor eliminations
of the system. To be sure, this is an equalizer
and would only act in that same force wherein
normal rest to the body becomes recuperative
powers for same. This, then, rather a preven-

tative of such conditions arising in the body
than of a curative force, save as the body
through mental forces, and through the action
of the normal forces, pertaining to appetite
and rebuilding forces of the body, would become
assistance to same.
"We are through for the present." 1800-4

"Mrs. C: You will have before you the reading
taken on July 27th, 1925, regarding battery
appliance. You will please answer the following
questions regarding this, as I ask them of you.
"Mr. C: Yes we have the information as given
regarding the battery appliance, as was given
on July 27, 1925 (1800-4) and we find this,
as has been given, would prove very beneficial
in any condition relating to the vibratory
forces in physical body, especially that of
first stages of rheumatism, catarrh, or any
condition that affects the system regarding
the eliminations for the body.
"This we find would be well that everyone use
such appliance, for the system would be improved in every condition that relates to the
body being kept in attunement, as it were,
for the forces as are exerted are such that
the body responds to those conditions as are
made by such an appliance, when constructed
in the way and manner as given. Thus:
"Using two pieces of carbon steel (plain, see?).
These will take the magnetic forces, or supply
magnetic forces the better than hardened or
tool steel, and these would be at least 4½"
to 5" in length. ¼" to 5/8" wide, with thick-
ness, of ¼" to ½", see? These incased in tin
or metal or rubber container, packed with
charcoal (plain), with carbon or insulation
between each. These then should have small
wire (copper-insulated) attached to each piece
of steel. In turn, small plates attached to
each end of the wire (loose, see?). This then
may be attached to the body. Under the regular

or normal conditions, attach one to each
extremity of body, to right and left side of
body. When any conditions relating to centra-
lization in body, attach one to the umbilicus,
or just above, or the right or left, depending
upon which side of the body is needing the
condition to be changed. The container, then,
should be placed always in water, with ice in
same. This may be kept on body for an indeter-
minate period, thirty to sixty minutes, giving
a change in the vibration of the body.
"These made, may be distributed to many people,
and be found very beneficial in any condition
as given. Do that.
"Q.- In cold weather, may the appliance just
be hung outside and then attached to the body?
"A.- Always placed in cold or ice water, for
the action of water on the elements produces
the vibration necessary for body.
"These we may find that, if there is the
necessity of such liquids being given the body
as stimulants of any nature; that is, of the
vibratory nature, or any drug or property that
is of the sympathetic nature, attached to the
negative pole, may add same to the vibration
of body in that degree as to be beneficial to
the body; such as Quinine, Gold, and Silver
Nitrate, Iodine, Spirits of Camphor. Any of
the elements carrying eighty-five or above
percent of alcohol. These would be made in
this manner.
"An attachment of Nickel, with a projection
that would protrude into such container. These
would be attached to the pole or wire, you
see, with the metal in the central portion of
same. This we find would gradually be carried,
or the effects of the vibration, to the system."
                                          1800-5
"Mr. C: Yes, we have the body and those conditions that surround same, (2096). This we
have had before. In many respects we find
conditions have been on the improve. While

there is the tendency for the body to immediately take on weight when the diet is neglected,
or too much sugars or too much starches are
added to the system, we will find that were
the vibrations added in the proper ratio or
manner from the Radio-Active Appliance, (the
plain) the assimilated forces will be better
distributed in the system and the vibrations
as are set up will be nearer equalized, and
that conditions will then continue to be in
a nearer normal way and manner: for these
vibrations now, with the changes as have come
about in the system, will act with the glands
of the system that tend to make for too much
of the avoirdupois of body." 2096-2

"...vibrations from the appliance given are
not just as talismanic conditions, nor are
they which operates through the imaginations
of a body, but when properly compounded or
constructed these correspond with the laws of
physics...While they are seemingly of little
or no use from outward appearance, their constructive forces are in an orderly manner...
This enables the quieting, then, from within,
and allows the forces to become predominant
that are constructive to vitality in system."
957-3
"The vibration are given off, which creates
that same vibration (within the system)... would
act as a Universal Force, as would be changed
according to the conditons of the system."
1800-6
"...with any condition that becomes abnormal
in the human body, it, the condition, is the
lack of an equilibrium produced by the lack
of that necessary to produce that vibration
in that portion of the organism of the human
body that becomes distressed or dis-eased..."
1800-10
"The Appliance's vibration" are the lowest
form of electrical forces that move as energies

from the etheronic forces--or of the lowest
form of static, or of the electrical creative
forces." 681-2

"...the application of the Radio-Active (appliance) is just the opposite end of electrical
forces which create that which is the basis
of life. For while electrical forces are life
in its activity, in man--save where they are
to destroy the plasms (sic) that work upon
the body itself--they are more helpful in the
low form than the high form." 680-1

"Just as a battery may be charged or discharged,
so may the human body be recharged by the
production of coordination (by) the Appliance."
                                        5428-1
Wet Cell Battery:

"Now, as to preparation of the Wet Cell Appliances, this would be the preferable manner
though, to be sure, these vary according to
the character of solution that in its radial
activity is to be conveyed to the body.
"These would be built in such a manner that
the container would hold at least a gallon and
a half of solution, see? But the container
would be at least half a gallon larger.
"Preferably such containers should be made of
a composition, or rubberoid that does not
break or become changed by the contraction
and expansion owing to the activity of the
solution in same. The top of the container
should preferably be of the same material, or
it may be of glass, or it may be of crockware
or of wood; preferably made to specifications
of a square or an oblong container that would
hold two gallons, see? marked or the measure-
ment given on same so that the gallon and a
half is indicated when the quantity of water
is put in same. The following ingredients make
up the activities of the solution in same:

    Willow Charcoal   ½ *pound*
    Copper Sulfate   1½ *pounds*
    Sulphuric Acid, C.P.I. 1 *ounce*

"Common Zinc (or pieces of zinc tin or zinc may be cut), 30 grams that will produce with the Acid, the Copper Sulfate, and the electrical vibrations.

"This would be the manner of preparation.

"The poles used would be half inch (½) rods, square or circular dependent upon which is the easier to procure. But make the specifications so that these are uniform; dependent, of course, upon whether the container is high or low, square or round, or what!

"One pole would be of Copper, the other Nickel.

"The Copper pole is always the positive, to which a Copper plate is attached.

"And the leads should be so attached that they may be long enough to prevent causing disturbance to the individual using same.

"A Nickel plate, larger, would be attached to the Nickel pole; always the negative, and would be that which would pass through a solution or go plain, dependent upon the order of same. This plate should be at least two and a half or three inches (2½ or 3") in diameter, circular; preferably made so that it is just a little bit cupped, so that the attachments to same would be on the back side and not on the edges. Those attachment would be fastened either by the countersinking and a hole, or by soldering or the projections on same so that these may be tied or the plates applied on any portion of the body, see?

"Both plates should be fixed in the same manner, though the Copper plate would not be larger than an inch (1") of the whole plate. But these should be made so they form a cup, or a sort of a roll, you see, so that the attachments make them directly in connection with the body itself; forming, as it were, a little vacuum under the plate where attached to the body.

"As to the preparation of a container into
which there would be put such solutions as
Camphor, Gold, Silver, Iodine, or any of the
preparations that are soluble in alcohol.

"We find that any of such solutions may be
given to the body, as we have indicated
through this manner; causing the activity of
same without it passing through the system
itself, for it may be directed to various
organs of the system that are in need of such
elements as to the glands in any portion of
the system that receive impulses from the
cerebro-spinal system, or from the sympathetic or the vegetable system, or from any of
the ganglia of the lymph or emunctory circulation that forms itself in portions of the
body.

"So as indicated, the attachments should be
prepared or made in a manner so that they are
encased over the centers where attached, in a
sort of cup shape, so as to draw or such as a
cup would.

"Then the container for such a solution (being
upon the longer lead, the Nickel, and attached
to the Nickel passing through the solution)
would be preferably of glass, preferably with
a metal, plastic or hard rubber top. Have it
so arranged that the lead which goes into same,
in the form of a U, may be taken entirely out,
see? and so that the ends of the wire that
attaches to same have tips on same, both to
the box and to the glass or container itself
in which the solution is put. Such a container
should be able to hold four to six (4 to 6)
ounces; preferably the six (6) ounce container.
Hence it would be such a shape and size as not
to be of an obtuse nature in handling. And
have the leads sufficiently long that they do
not cause the solution to swing in space in
its connection, you see. These should be at
least four feet long, or three feet from the
container to the body or more.

"These are the specifications:
"As to what is to be used in these, this will
be indicated in such information as may be
supplied for the body itself.
"Make these in conformity to these specifications and they will be proper.
"As to the preparation for the teeth, the gums,
the mouth in Ipsab:
"This would be made to those specifications
as indicated. The only condition about which
there has been any question, as we find, is
as to being sure that each quantity of the
water the saline solution or ocean water is
of the same volatile measure (or specific
gravity) when it is used, see? If this does
not come to the same specific gravity, add
common salt to make same. The specific gravity
of sea water should be one and seven-tenths.
                                    1800-25
"EC: Yes, Here we have quite a disturbance
with this body, (3976). This (disturbance) is
of a karmic nature. It is as much or more (a
lesson) for those responsible for the body--
as well as for the learning of patience by the
body itself.
"...Thus the treatments here would be best
given by the mother--that is, in the present
circumstances.
"Use the low electrical vibrations from the
Wet Cell Appliance carrying into the system
vibratorially the properties of Chloride of
Gold to build nerve energy and to coordinate
the relations of the cerebro-spinal, the
sympathetic and the sensory organism. The
proportions would be one grain Chloride of
Gold Sodium, to each ounce of distilled water
and use three ounces of the Solution for each
charge; renewing the Solution every fifteen
days. Every thirty days renew the charge
for the Appliance. The small plate would be
attached to three different centers alternately. The Appliance would be used for thirty

minutes each day; one day attaching the small
plate to the 3rd cervical, the next day to the
9th dorsal, and the next day to the 4th lumbar.
Be sure to rotate the attachments in this
order.
"These are the three centers through which
there is the activity of the kundaline forces
that act as suggestions to the spiritual forces
for distribution through the seven centers of
the body.
"Use that period of suggestions to the body.
Though there may not be the hearing, there may
not be the perfect vision, there may not be
the normal taste, the normal voice, we find
that the soul, the entity, the subconscious,
the unconscious and the superconsciousness
will respond--by the continued drum of the
suggestion given. Use the mother's own words,
but this is as the purpose of such a prayer
or suggestion:
"MAY THIS BODY BE SO ATTUNED TO THE INFINITE
THAT IT MAY BE PREPARED HERE AND NOW FOR THE
GREATER SERVICE THAT IT MAY RENDER TO ITS FEL-
LOW MAN IN THIS EXPERIENCE."
"Do that.
"We are through with this reading." 3676-1

Therefore:

"Use the periods when the....Appliance is
attached as a period not of conversation but
rather of contemplation and meditation, as
periods in which the body will review its own
experiences in the earth, its relationships
and that the body is planning to do with its
life in relationships to others, and as to
the reasons for the body being in the material
experience in the present and what it intends
to do with the opportunities for being an expression of its ideal in this sojourn."

                                        4030-1
"And use that period, when the Appliance is

attached, for meditation; when the body would
meditate upon its purposes in the earth, its
thanks and praise to the living God; its
desires to be the channel for a blessing, for
a helpful experience; for the knowledge of God
in the life and experience of others."

2800-1

"With the Appliance and with the meditative
forces that make for concentration, the body
will be enabled to fit itself physically and
mentally to be of a greater service, to find
more and greater opportunities for the expression of that gained..." 531-6

"Q.- Is the Radio-Active Appliance working
properly, and should it be used?
"A.- This used keeps a normal balance and is
most effective for resting, and is a good aid
when meditation is desirable.
"For as we find, the body is as a triune. As
the Father, the Son, the Holy Spirit, so the
body, the mind, the soul. If they are as one
--body, mind, soul--as the effective activity
of a low current of electrical reaction or
radiation is created in the active forces of
the Radio-Active Appliance--it brings to the
system just those influences; the tendency to
make the body-physical, the body-mental and
the mental-spiritual forces more and more in
accord by a unison.
"Hence in the use of this, use these as the
periods of thy meditations, and in thy reading
of the Scriptures that refer to thee. Read
them not as history, read them not as axioms
or as dogmas, but as of thine own being. For
in the study of these ye will find that ye draw
unto that force from which the writers of same
gained their strength, their patience.
"And as He hath given, in learning patience,
as all do in suffering, ye become aware of
your soul and its relationships to the Creative
Forces that were experienced by the writers

*of almost all of our history of same; and so
these are ever this:*
*"He is the same yesterday, today and forever.
And as has been their experience, not possibly
in the same manner but each to his own calling.
For some are ministers, some are healers, some
are preachers. But to all is given according
to the measure of their faith. (Ex. 28)*
*"And as ye apply this, though a mechanical
implement made by man--yet also was the ephod
also was the altar made by man--yet these have
brought, these may bring, these do bring, even
as the vision of the Cross, even as Gethsemane's
garden, even as the ordinances have their place
in the awakening of the consciousness of the
inner bring of a soul, of a man, so may this be
--not as a rosary, not as a picture, but rather
as uniting the body, mind, the soul with that
trinity--God, the Father, the Son, the Spirit.*
*"Thus may it bring to thee those experiences
that are thine alone. And again He has given,
'We have much work for (1173) to do.'"1173-8*

The object of this chapter is simply to satisfy
the mind of the reader that there is a philosophy back
of the utility of the Appliances, which experience
proves is able to develop an attainment of personal
balance and harmony not otherwise enjoyed. It is the
product of actual experience. The theories concerning
the result may not be understood, but the benefits
that have accompanied this course of application are
beyond the reach of doubt.

Nevertheless, the finger of science has been
pointing too long in the direction of the theory of
the Appliances to vary much from the meridian of truth.
While it is in a practical sense unnecessary, yet we
believe it will be interesting to every one to glance
briefly over the panorama that covers so much of the
history of humanity relative to Electro-Therapy.

The brief view we have taken of electricity show
us a wonderful talent force permeating all things, and
in our own bodies, evidently under the control of the

will. The known laws of this force does teach us the possibility of the mutual influence between portions of the body, in proportion to their differences of electrical density and environment. Every part of the system not in good electrical contact with another, polarizes itself and its neighbors. Under such favoring conditions the tension of this polarity may leap all bounds and set up an interchange of dynamic electricities. Some of these inducing elements are: a greater difference of density between the parts; sufficient approximation to reduce the resistance of the conductors, and a vibration of the part itself; as, for instance, would be perfectly secured by a full resonant force in action and reaction.

We know that persons affect us differently; some soothe, while others excite us. This influence varies according to the time, place and weather, and is most evidently in accordance with our very own electrical condition, or, as we familiarly say, "our health." Undoubtedly much of this is directly the result of electrical disturbance within us, and is therefore very similar to the activity of the parts within the system.

We find that in addition to the well known ordinary electricity in our bodies, which seems to act independently of our wishes, there is a similar force that seems to be related directly to our volition, and is yet distinct from the electrical fluid that accompanies every muscular action.

The force now in question is one that manifests electrical phenomena on external objects when the mind so intends. This force can be directly internally to any part or organ of the body in a similar fashion. Doubtless this is mainly the purpose of the Appliances, to direct the force to areas that are insufficiently supplied or where there exists a blockage. It transfers energy from one section to another, that is, from one abundantly supplied to one that is lacking, and operates similarly as will-power which can be directed toward any organ or set of organs in the body.

The following readings regarding the transfering of this energy are direct and to the point.

"In the Radio-Active (Appliance) the body builds the charge to be discharged through the instrument into other portions of the body."
                                        1800-28

"(The Appliance) may be called the magnet that builds up...So the discharge then (that builded up) is constantly to the opposite extremity to which the Appliance is (first) attached."
                                        1179-3

"For, as the vibrations are controlled through the activity of the Radio-Active Appliance, this takes energies in portions of the body, builds up and discharges body electrical energies that revivify portions of the body where there is a lack of energies stored."
                                        3105-1

"There is nothing in the Appliance of itself. For, know, as you are told in the Book, in the law--all that is within heaven and earth, as well as hell, is within the body of the living individual. To cause same to respond to those vibration cells of creative energies, so that each corpuscle of the building, of the staying or of the resisting variety, is aware of its purpose to renew itself, may best be attained from its own source of supply--which is within. "The activity of the Appliance, then, is to build that low form of energy (which is electrical in itself) as to build up in the one extremity and discharge in the other."3119-1

Undoubtedly, the recommendation of Cayce to be in a prayerful or in a meditative attitude so enables this constructive or Creative Force to be much more expressive in its activity. There is a need for more research in this area, for the possibilities exist and certainly are tremendous in helping to solve the ailments of a sick and ailing society.

CHAPTER TWENTY-TWO

TRUE SCOPE OF MEDICINE

Any one able to read the signs of the times cannot help observing the powerful influence which the natural healing philosophy is already exerting upon the trend of modern medical science.

On the rank and file the idea of drugless healing has about the same effect as a red flag on a mad bull. There are still very few physicians in general practice today who would not lose their bread and butter if they attempted to practice drugless healing on their patients. Both the profession and the public will need a good deal more education along the natural healing lines before they will see the light.

It seems many of those who have adopted natural methods of living and of treating ailments have acquired an actual horror of the practices of modern medicine. However, this extreme attitude is not justified. It also appears that many are under the impression that the natural healing followers condemn the use of any and all medicines. This, however, is not so.

The use of drugs are condemned in so far as they are poisonous and destructive, and in so far as they suppress acute diseases or healing crises, which are nature's cleansing and healing efforts; but on the other hand it is realized that there is a wide field for the helpful application of medicinal remedies in so far as they act as foods to the tissues of the body and as the neutralizers and eliminators of waste and morbid materials.

Examples as given in the readings:

"For the eliminations generally, we would use Zilatone as an activity upon the eliminative system, so that the organs of the system may be cleansed throughout. Half an hour after the morning meal take one Zilatone Tablet: half

an hour to an hour after the noon meal take
another; then in the evening about 2 hours
after the meal, take 2 tablets. And then leave
off for at least 2 or 3 days, before this may
be repeated again." 1523-1

"Then we would increase the eliminations to
carry away more of the poisons and toxins from
the system. For this body in the present, and
with the (work) activities, we would use the
mineral rather than the vegetable eliminants,
especially such as may be found in Upjohn's
citrocarbonates. This we would take--a heaping
teaspoonful each morning before any meal is
taken. Let it effervesce, and drink a full
glass of water with the spoonful dissolved in
same, and then another glass of water afterwards. Do drink more water." 2051-6

"For a laxative take Senna Leaf (Senna Pod)
tea, using 4 or 5 of the leaves place in an
empty cup, and then pour hot water on it and
let stand for 30 minutes to 45 minutes; strain
and drink it. Do this about once a week and it
will be good for the body, as it does not become
habit-forming and is a correct laxative for
most individuals--though not everyone." 457-1

"Begin with broken doses of Castoria or with
Caldwell's Syrup of Pepsin--Senna of Fig Base.
Half a teaspoonful every hour until good eliminations are set up.
"The Castoria formula has been changed and is
not as complete as the Syrup of Pepsin; hence
the suggestion for the Pepsin as a substitute."
                                        2824-4
"We would give the Castoria in broken doses,
ten to twelve drops every half hour until there
are thorough eliminations." 2824-5

"Now to cleanse the system, we would set up
eliminations with Castoria." 2572-5

To every form of chronic disease there exists in the system, on the one hand, an excess of certain morbid materials, and on the other hand, a deficiency of certain mineral constituents, organic salts, which are essential to the normal functions of the body.

Thus, in all anemic diseases the blood is lacking in iron, which picks up the oxygen from the air cells of the lungs and carries it into the tissues, and in sodium, which combines with the carbonic acid (coal gas) that is constantly being liberated in the system and conveys it to the organs of depuration, especially the lungs and the skin. In point of fact, oxygen starvation is due in a much greater degree to the deficiency of sodium and the consequential accumulation of carbonic acid in the system (carbonic acid asphyxia), than to the lack of iron in the blood, as assumed by the regular school of medicine.

Foods or medicinal remedies which will supply this deficiency of iron and sodium in the organism will tend to overcome the anemic condition.

The great range of uric acid diseases, such as rheumatism, arterio-sclerosis, and certain forms of diabetes are due, on the other hand, to the excessive use of acid-producing foods, and on the other hand, to a deficiency in the blood of certain alkaline mineral elements, especially sodium, magnesium, and potassium, whose office it is to neutralize and eliminate the acids which are created and liberated in the processes of starchy and protein digestion.

Any foods or medicines which will provide the system with sufficient quantities of the acid-binding, alkaline mineral salts will prove to be good medicine for all forms of acid diseases.

The mineral constituents necessary to the vital economy of the organism should, however, be supplied in the organic form.

From what has been said, it becomes apparent that it is impossible to draw a sharp line of distinction between foods and medicines. All foods which serve the above named purpose are good medicines, and all non-poisonous herb extracts, homeopathics, vito-chemical remedies that have the same effect upon the system are for the same reason, good foods.

But it is quite possible that, through continued abuse, the digestive apparatus has become so weak and so abnormal that it cannot function properly, that it cannot absorb and assimilate from the natural foods a sufficient quantity of the elements which the organism needs. In such cases it may be very helpful and, indeed, imperative to take some medicinal properties that have the required mineral elements and salts in organic combinations which are easily assimilated.

Foremost among these food-medicines we find prescribed in the Edgar Cayce readings. These remedies contain in organic form the physiological salts that are needed by the organism for the ordinary functional activities of the body as well as for the neutralization and elimination of disease poisons.

Cayce accomplishes in his psychic laboratory, by chemical processes, what nature does in the vital processes of the vegetable kingdom; he prescribes organic mineral combinations which are suited best to each individual's needs, to the plane of vegetable life itself.

The homeopathic medicaments, as fully explained at length in a previous chapter, produce their good results not because of the dosage but because they work in harmony with the laws of nature.

Cayce never hesitated, therefore, to prescribe for individuals homeopathic medicines, herb decoctions and extracts, and the vito-chemical remedies which assists in the elimination of morbid matter from the system and in building up blood and lymph on a normal basis, that is, remedies which supply the organism with the mineral elements in which it is deficient in the organic, easily assimilable forms. Herein lies the legitimate scope of medicinal remedies.

"Q.- What medicines should he take?
"A.- This will depend upon the general elimi-
nations or the general activity. The less
medications, as medicines, the better it will
be for the body; provided these are not neces-
sary to add stimulation to some depleted or

defunct activity of an organ or for the strengthening of the body in some way or manner. But these are rather as tonics and stimulants than as medications, as we find. For nature should be the healer." 1173-5

"Let these be some considerations: If there is the constant dosage or constant application of synthetic influences, these become at times hindrances to the body. But if there are those activities from nature's storehouse, then we find these work with the Creative Energies and impulses of an organism to create and to bring about coordinating influences in the system."
1173-8

"...though there are characters that may be absorbed through the application of medical natures; yet the general condition, as a whole --this is broadly speaking--when there are properties given that destroy, or dry, or cause that of eliminations, these are at the expense of some other portion of the system. The osteopathic nature of treatment is, in the greatest measure, to aid the physical forces in the human body to adjust themselves, through the continued keeping in accord the various conditions as respecting the eliminations in the system." 264-4

"These (proper eliminations through alimentary canal, respiratory system, kidneys, liver, perspirations) may best be brought about by the manipulations osteopathically. That's why the osteopathic profession should stand at the head for most of physical ailments and treatments; for the general distribution--when properly administered (it may be bungled, of course)--properly administered--it aids most in coordination with the general eliminations and corrective measures where lesions, adhesions or such conditions arise, and operates through normalcy; and so when conditions are

*adjusted, the body is near normal and not.
overtaxed in one portion, as are in so many--
either as purely adjustments or that of medication that operates at the expense of another
vibratory force set up."* 325-28

*"Now, to meet the needs of these conditions
in this body, it becomes necessary, as we see,
then, to create the correct vibration, and
remove from the body these conditions in the
normal way, without disturbing the equilibrium
of the functioning of any organ above or below
in its (the organ's) normal condition. Or, we
produce the change of the condition in various
portions of the body, as indications show that
different parts are disturbed at the present
time. To keep the circulation in the correct
vibration, not medicine in the system, for
these would be as those that would disturb one
portion by excess at the expense of another
portion of the body, but we would create that
correct vibration that will bring about the
normal forces to each portion, and especially
stimulating the blood supply to that condition
wherein it (the blood supply) may be kept
nearer normal throughout, and at all times.
"Then, we would apply to the solar plexus
center those vibrations as are found in the
Radium Appliance, and this will, as we see,
act to the system in this manner.
"In that vibration as is set in motion by these,
is to clarify the blood stream, through the
ability of each cellular force to function in
its normal manner, by being brought to its
highest vibration that will function with each
portion of the system through which it passes.
Hence, acting not only as a strainer, but as
a rejuvenator to each center through which the
blood stream--in this perfect vibration--is
sent."* 121-1

Once again:

*"Then, to bring about a more normal condition
for this body, and bring the relief to many
portions of the system, would be first to give
that correction as is necessary through the
deep manipulation and the adjustments, osteopathically, of those conditions along the
cerebro-spinal system, cleansing the blood at
the same time by the use of the Alpine or Rino
ray, given at least twice each week. The
osteopathic adjustments should be at least
twice each week, or each day at first for one
week, and then twice each week." 86-1*

*"For as is understood by the meaning of osteo-
pathic treatments, these are not what might
be termed as curative forces; they are those
applications that RELEASE energies that are
in the body-forces. And the natural tendency
is for each each organ, each cellular force,
to do its proper activity towards the correlating of the whole. Thus it is as much of a
preventative application or treatment as it
is curative." 1467-17*

*"As a system of treating human ills, osteopathy
--WE would give--is more beneficial than most
measures that may be given. Why? In any preventative or curative measure, that condition
to be produced is to assist the system to gain
its normal equilibrium. It is known that each
organ receives impulses from other portions
of the system by the suggestive forces (sympathetic nervous system) and by circulatory
forces (the cerebro-spinal system and the blood
supply itself). These course through the system
in very close parallel activity in EVERY single
portion of the body.*
*"Hence stimulating ganglia from which impulses
arise--either sympathetically or functionally
--must then be helpful in the body gaining an
equilibrium." 902-1*

Medicinal properties:

"Then to give the relief to this body, and bring about the nearer equilibrium, we would give into the system, taking exercises of a specific nature for the whole system:
"To one gallon of rain water, we would add:

Sarsaparilla Root	2 ounces
Burdock Root	2 ounces
Yellow Dock Root	2 ounces
Yellow Root	2 ounces
Black Snake Root	2 ounces
Buchu Leaves	10 grains
Elder Flower	4 ounces

"Reduce by simmering (not boiling) to one quart. Strain while warm and add three drams of Balm of Gilead and four ounces of grain alcohol, using the buds, you see, in the Gilead.
"The dose would be a teaspoonful four times each day.
"The exercise would be for that portion of the body that is under stress at each time the body should take the exercise, which is night and mornings. At times we will find this shifted from the abdomen to the pelvis, again to the extremities, again to the limbs and shoulders. Each should be exercised in the manner as to give the release of the tissues and muscular forces of that portion of the body. Make, specifically, the body take quantities of water. Take this as medicinal propertise. The body does not drink sufficient water." 26-1

"Now, to give relief to this body—and to give the normal action of the system, would be to give that in the system that will produce the perfect elimination, to give the incentives to the intestinal tract to relieve this portion of the body from having, or being possessed with, auto-intoxication, as is the case at times as we find here; and to give to the nerve

centers, that is, will give, the correct incentives to all the muscular and lymph forces,
for there is little lymph in the system--take
this in the body:
"To one gallon of distilled water, we would add:

Wild Cherry Bark	2 ounces
Prickly Ash Bark	2 ounces
Black Snake Root	2 ounces
Yellow Dock Root	2 ounces
Mandrake Root	3 grains
Elder Flower	2 ounces

"Simmer, not boil, until reduced to one quart;
strain; while warm add six ounces of grain
alcohol with three drams of Balsam of Tolu. The
dose would be a teaspoonful four times each
day just before meals and just before retiring.
"Each evening the body should take exercises
just before taking the dose of medicine last,
you see." 95-1

"Then, to meet the needs of the conditions in
this body: This wiil require that activity
both in a systematic, in a sympathetic, and
in an action that will be consistent and
persistent to bring the better condition for
the body. With same, we will find the rest of
the natural life in this experience will be
more plesant in its reactions and activity
than has been the first half of it.
"First, then, we will begin with that as will
be necessary for the basis of the changes as
are to be brought about in the physical functioning of the body--though we will find it
will be necessary in every six to eight weeks
that a change be made in the administrations
as the basis of that to be accomplished for,
in, through, and by the active functioning
forces of this body to be brought to normalcy.
"We begin, then, with that of the constitutional, and this should be used for at least
ten days to two weeks before other applications
of any nature are given. With the use of these,

discontinue those of the effect that have been
used and are being used at times.

"Prepare the basis, or the carrier, as this:
To ½ gallon of distilled water, add Wild Cherry
Bark, 6 ounces. Reduce by slow boiling (retain-
ing the steam in same) to half the quantity.
Then add 4 ounces of beet sugar, first dissolved
in 2 ounces of distilled or plain water. Then
reduce at least to ½ the quantity again, see?
Then we would add:

Compound Syrup of Sarsaparilla	1 ounce
Essence or tincture of Stillingia	¼ ounce
Essence of Silkweed	½ ounce
10% solution Iodide of Potassium	¼ ounce
10% solution Bromide of Potassium	½ ounce
Essence of, or Tincture of	
Elder Flower	¼ ounce

"Then add 2 drams Balsam of Tolu cut in 2
ounces grain alcohol. Shake solution together
before the dose is taken, which should be a
teaspoonful half an hour before meals."109-1

"To give balance in the system, necessary to
meet resistive forces, and to overcome, we
would add to the system, they which will assist
in producing the elimination through the whole
system the building to assist the blood rebuilding forces. Take this into the system:
"To one gallon of rain water, or distilled
water we would add:

Sarsaparilla Root	4 ounces
Wild Cheery Bark	2 ounces
Black Root	2 ounces
Mandrake Root	20 grains

"This should be simmered, not boiled, until
reduced to one quart. Strain while warm. Add
four ounces of grain alcohol, with three drams
of Balsam Of Tolu. The dose would be a tablespoonful half hour before meals of evening.

"The body should have vibrations, of electric
vibration, electrically driven, not the electricity itself, over the whole length of the

*spine from the first cervical to the end of
the spine, the across the body at the sacral
plexus, and down the sciatic nerve to the knees.
"By the time the second quantity of this is
taken, the body will feel the difference in
the condition, and be able to digest the foods,
which should not be meats, but rather of the
coarser--and vegetable matter, taking or using
whole wheat as gruel. Do that." 159-1*

Atomidine:

     Iodine, as most people know it, is a solution or
tincture used as an antiseptic and is a non-metallic
chemical element in molecular form. Through independent
research aided by the readings from Edgar Cayce, a
new form of Iodine was developed, that is, a solution
which carries Iodine in atomic form. Is distributed
commercially as an antiseptic, and is recommended in
the physical readings of Cayce for those individuals
in need of a "purifier and stabilizer" for an endocrine
gland activity. The warning is made that no other form
of medicines or any alcohol be taken internally when
taking Atomodine, although external applications may
not require this precaution.

*"As we find, there is a lack of activity of
the glands in the thyroid areas. This causes
a weakness in the activities to nails and hair
over the body.
"We would take small doses of Atomidine to
purify the thyroid activity. Take one drop
each morning for five days in succession. Then
leave off for five days.
"Do use the diets that carry Iodine in their
natural forms. Use only kelp salt or deep sea
salt. Plenty of seafoods. These are preferable
for the body. Not too much sweets. The egg
yolk but not the white of egg should be taken."*
                                          4056-1
*"As we find, there are conditions causing
disturbance with this body. These are because*

*of improper coordination of the activities of
the inner and outer glandular forces as related
to the thyroid. This allows for deficiencies
in certain chemical forces, especially as is
related to the epidermis, or the activities
in the toes and the fingers and the hair.
These are distressing disturbances to the
body.* ·

*"There is that which has caused much of the dis-
turbance—a long standing subluxation existent in the 3rd and 4th lumbar centers, which
prevents the perfect circulation through the
glands of the thyroid area.*

*"We would make corrections osteopatically in
that specific area, coordinating the 3rd cervical and the lumbar axis with same.*

*"We would also begin taking Atomidine internal-
ly as a purifier for the glands and to stimulate
better thyroid activity. This may change the
heart's regularity for the time but if it is
properly administered and the osteopathic
corrections are made properly, we will find
changes wrought in the activities in the epidermis and as associated or related to the hair.*

3904-1

*"Q.- How to prevent tooth decay which I've had
an awful lot of the past three years.*

*"A.- Have them attended to, and add to the
system occassionally—Atomodine as a manner of
gaining better control of the activity of the
glands which formulate the circulation through
teeth and structural portion of the body. One
drop 5 days at a time and then skip 2 weeks.
Then again—do this throughout a whole year,
and you'll have your teeth in very good fix if
local attention is given the rest."* 5313-4

*"For four or five days it would be well to
take internally two drops of the Atomidine
full or commercial strength, see, in half a
glass of water. Then, be precautious as to the
diet, in the general manner as we have indicated
for the body."* 261-33

All medical properties which build up the system on a normal natural basis and increases its fighting power against disease without in any way inflicting injury upon the organism are welcome adherents to the natural healing methods of treatment.

On the other hand, Cayce did not prescribe the use of any drugs or medicines with which to hinder, check, or suppress nature's cleansing and regenerating processes. He never prescribed anything in the least degree poisonous. He avoided all manner of prescription drugs. A judicious diet, cold-water application and, if necessary, warm-water injections of colonics for cases of constipation will all do what is claimed for poisonous drugs.

For many years past, physicians of the different schools of medicine, diet experts, and food chemists have been divided on the question of whether or not mineral substances which in the organic form enter into the composition of the human body may safely be used in foods and medicines in the organic form.

The medical profession holds almost unanimously that this is permissable and good practice, so that nearly every allopathic medical prescription contains some such inorganic substance, or worse than that, one or more virulent mineral poisons, such as phosphorus, mercury, arsenic, etc.

So far, the discussion about the usefulness, or harmfulness of inorganic materials as foods and as medicines was largely theorical and mostly controversial to say the least. Neither party had any positive proof for its contention.

But nature's records in the iris of the eye settle the question once and for all. One of the fundamental principles of the science of Eye Diagnosis is that nothing shows in the iris by abnormal signs or discolorations except that which is abnormal in the body or injurious to it. When substances which are most uncogenial or poisonous to the system accumulate in any part or organ of the human organism in sufficient quantities, they will indicate their presence by certain signs and abnormal colors in the corresponding areas of the iris.

In this way nature makes known by her records in the eye what substances are injurious to the body, and which are harmless.

Certain mineral elements, such as iron, sodium, potassium, lime, magnesium, phosphorus, sulphur, and others, which are among the important constituents of the human body, may be taken in the organic form as found in fruits and vegetables, or in herb extracts and the vito-chemical remedies, in large amounts, in fact, far beyond the actual needs of the body, but they do not show in the iris of the eye, because they are easily eliminated from the system.

"Q.- Please give the foods that would supply these (minerals).
"A.- We have given them; cereals that carry the heart of the grain, vegetables of the leafy kind, fruits and nuts as indicated. The almond carries more phosphorus and iron in a combination easily assimilated than any other nut"
1131-2

"So keep an excess of foods that carry especially vitamin B, iron and such. Not that the concentrated form, you see, but obtain these from the foods. These would include all fruits, all vegetables that are yellow." 1968-7

"As to the diet: Add to the diet more of those foods that carry vitamin B_1. In conjunction with the applications we have suggested for improvement, it is preferable that this be done by taking an excess of foods carrying same than by taking the vitamins in concentrated form as in tablets or capsule." 2564-1

"Let the iron be rather taken in the foods (instead of from medicinal sources) as it is more easily assimilated from the vegetable forces...." 1187-9

"The phosphorus-forming foods are principally carrots, lettuce (rather the leaf lettuce,

which has more soporific activity than the head lettuce), shell fish, salsify, the peelings of Irish potatoes (if they are not too large), and things of such nature....Citrusfruit juices, and plenty of milk--the Bulgarian (buttermilk is) the better, or the fresh milk that is warm with the animal heat which carries more of the phosphorus and more of those activities that are less constipating, or acting more with the lacteals and the ducts of the liver, the kidneys and the bowels themselves."

560-2

Therefore:

"Supply in the vital energies that which ye call vitamins or elements. For remember, though we may give many combinations there are only four elements in your body: salt, water, soda and iodine. These are the basic elements; they make all the rest! Each vitamin, as a component part of an element, is simply a combination of these other influences--given a name, mostly for confusion, by those who would tell you what to do for a price." 2533-6

"What are those elements in food or drink that give growth or strength to the body? Vitamins! What are vitamins? The Creative Forces working with the body energies for the renewing of the body." 3511-1

"Q.- What relation do the vitamins bear to the glands? Give specific vitamins affecting specific glands.
"A.- You want a book written on these!
"They are food for same. Vitamins are that from which the glands take those necessary influences to supply the energies to enable the varied organs of the body to reproduce themselves. Would it ever be considered that your toenails would be reproduced by the same (gland) as would supply the breast, the head,

or the face? Or that the cuticle would be
supplied from the same source as would supply
the organ of the heart itself? These are taken
from glands that control the assimilated foods
and hence the necessary elements or vitamins
in same to supply the various forces for
enabling each organ, each functioning of the
body to carry on in its creative or generative
forces, see?

"These begin with A--that supplies portions of
the nerves, to bone, to the brain force itself;
not all of this, but this is a part of A.

"B and B_1 supply the ability of the energies,
or the moving forces of the nerve and of the
white blood supply, as well as the white nerve
energy in the nerve force itself, the brain
for itself, and the ability of the sympathetic
or involuntary reflexes through the body. Now
this includes all, whether you are wiggling
your toes or your ears or batting your eye,
or what! In these we have that supplying to
the chyle that ability for it to control the
influence of fats, which is necessary (and
this body has never had enough of it to carry
on the reproducing of the oils that prevent
the tenseness in the joints, or that prevent
the joints from becoming atrophied or dry, or
to creak. At times the body has had some creaks!

"In C we find that which supplies the necessary
influences to the flexes of every nature
throughout the body, whether of a muscular or
tendon nature, or a heart reaction, or a kidney
contraction, or the liver contraction, or the
opening or shutting of your mouth, the batting
of the eye, or the supplying of the saliva and
the muscular forces in the face. These are all
supplied by C--not that it is the only supply,
but a part of same. It is that from which the
structural portions of the body are stored,
and drawn upon when it becomes necessary. And
when...(lack of C) becomes detrimental, or
there is a deficiency of same--which has been

> *for this body; it is necessary to supply same*
> *in such proportions as to aid; else the con-*
> *ditions become such that there are bad elimi-*
> *nations from the incoodination of the excretory*
> *functioning of the alimentary canal, as well*
> *as the heart, liver, and lungs, through the*
> *expelling of those forces that are a part of*
> *the structural portion of the body.* "G_{10}
> *supplies the general energies, or the sympa-*
> *thetic forces, of the body itself.*
> *"These are the principles."* 2072-9

In continuing, that if, however, the same minerals are taken in the inorganic form in any quantity, the iris will exhibit certain well-defined signs and discolorations in the areas corresponding to those parts of the body in which the minerals have accumulated.

Obviously, nature does not intend that all these mineral elements should enter the organism in the inorganic form, and so, therefore, the organs of depuration are not able to neutralize and eliminate them.

Thus, for instance, any amount of iron taken in vegetables or herb extracts, or in the vito-chemical remedies, will not be seen in the eye. Whatever is taken in excess of the needs of the body will promptly be eliminated.

If, however, similar quantities of iron are taken for the same length of time in the inorganic, mineral form, the iron will accumulate in the tissues of the stomach and bowels, and begin to show in the iris in the form of a rust-brown discoloration in the corresponding area of the digestive organs, directly around the pupil.

In a similar manner sodium, which is one of the most important mineral elements in the human body, if taken in the inorganic form, will show in a heavy, white rim along the outer edge of the iris. Sulphur will show in the form of yellowish discolorations in the area of the stomach and bowels. Iodine as in the medicinal, inorganic form, prepared from the ash of sea-weeds shows in the iris as well-defined, bright red spots. Phosphorus appears in whitish streaks and clouds in the areas corresponding to the organs in which it has accumulated.

An interesting exception to this rule is our own common table salt (Sodium Chloride), which is of an inorganic mineral combination. So far, the diagnosticians of the eyes have not discovered any sign in the iris for it. There seems to be something in its nature that makes it akin to organic substances, or like other inorganic minerals and their combinations they will show up in the iris.

This might explain why salt is the only inorganic mineral substance which is extensively used as food by humanity in general. Also animals who, guided by their natural instincts, are the finest discriminators in the selection of foods and medicines, do not hesitate to take salt freely (saltlicks) when they would not touch any other inorganic mineral.

Nevertheless, we do not wish to encourage the excessive use of salt, either in the cooking of food or at the table. Taken in considerable quantities, it is undoubtedly injurious to the tissues of the body.

Before the days of canned goods, scorbut or scurvy was a common disease among mariners and other people who had to subsist for long periods of time on salted meats and were deprived of raw fresh vegetables. The disease manifested as a breaking-down of the gums and other tissues of the body, accompanied by bleeding and much soreness. And as soon as these people partook of fresh fruits and vegetables, the scurvy disappeared.

The minerals contained in these organic salts (vitamins) foods furnished the building stones which imparted textile strength to the tissues and stopped the disintegration of the fleshy structure.

The natural healing regimen aims also to provide sodium chloride as well as the other basic mineral elements and salts required by the body in the organic form as exists in foods and natural medicines.

When the use of inorganic minerals is discontinued and when the proper methods of eliminative treatment, dietetic and otherwise, are applied, these mineral substances are gradually dislodged and carried out of the system. Simultaneously with their eliminations disappears the parallel signs in the iris of the eye and the disease symptoms which their presence had so created in the human organism.

In this connection it is a significant fact that those minerals which are congenial to the system, that is, those which in their organic state enter into the composition of the body, are that much more easily eliminated, if they have been taken in the inorganic form, than those substances which are naturally foreign and poisonous to the human organism, such as Mercury, Arsenic, Iodine, the Bromides, the different coal-tar preparations, etc.

This is proved by the fact that the signs of the minerals which are normal constituents of the human body, disappear from the iris of the eye much more quickly than the signs of those minerals which are foreign and naturally poisonous to the system.

The difficulty we experience in the eliminating of mineral poisons from the body would seem to indicate that nature never intended them to be used as foods or medicines. The intestines, kidneys, skin, mucous membranes, and other organs of depuration are evidently not constructed or prepared to cope with inorganic, poisonous substances and to eliminate them completely. Accordingly, these poisons show the tendency to accumulate in certain parts or organs of the body for which they have a special affinity, and then to act as the malicious irritants and destructive corrodents that they are.

The diseases which are the most difficult to cure even by the most radical application of the natural methods, are cases of drug poisoning. Substances which are foreign to the human organism, and especially the inorganic, mineral poisons, positively destroys the tissues and organs, and are much harder to eliminate from the system than the encumbrances of the morbid materials and waste matter produced in the organism itself, by wrong habits of living only. The obvious reason for this is that our organs of elimination are intended and constructed to execrete only such waste products as are formed in the organism in the process of metabolism.

THE IMPORTANCE OF A NATURAL DIET

While certain medicinal remedies in organic form may be very useful in supplying quickly a deficiency of mineral elements or vitamins in the system, we should aim to keep our bodies in a normal and healthy condition by proper food selection and in the right combinations. A brief outline of this will be found in the chapter on Dietetics.

Undoubtedly, nature has supplied all the elements which the human organism needs in abundance and in the right proportions in the natural foods, otherwise she would be a very ignorant organizer and provider.

We should all learn to select and combine food elements in such a manner that they supply all the needs of the body in the best possible way, and thus insure perfect health and strength without the use of drugs and other similar so called medicines.

Why should an attempt be made to cure anemia with inorganic iron, hyper-acidity of the stomach with baking soda, swollen glands with drugs, the itch with sulphur, rachitic conditions as in infants with lime water, etc., etc., when these mineral elements are contained in abundance and live, in organic form in fruits and vegetables and herbs, as well as in the vito-chemical remedies?

Unfortunately, however, a great many individuals, through wrong habits of living and of treating their aliments, have ruined their digestive organs to such an extent that they are incapable of properly assimilating their food and require, at least temporarily, stimulative treatment by natural methods and a supply of the indispensable organic mineral salts through medicinal food preparations.

In such cases the mineral elements must be provided in the most easily assimilable form, as in that of vegetable extracts (which should be prepared fresh every day), and in the vito-chemical remedies.

What has been said is sufficient, I believe, to justify the attitude of the natural healing school towards medicines in general. It explains why we should avoid the use of inorganic minerals and all poisonous substances, while on the other hand we find a wide and useful field of medicinal remedies contained in the form of blood and tissue of the body itself.

"But nature's storehouse (thine own body) may be induced to create every influence necessary for bringing greater and better and nearer normal conditions, if the hindrances are removed." 1309-1

"For as the body is the storehouse of all influences and forces from without, it has the abilities for the creating--with the correct firing or fuel for the body--that which is able to sustain, not only sustain but to recuperate and to rebuild, revitalize, regenerate the activities of the body." 1334-1

"...for the system can, and does create within itself all necessary either to cure or to sustain the virility of a body. Only when the system becomes so unbalanced as to need outside forces to create a different element of consciousness in the system is it necessary for medicinal properties or medicines for the body." 331-1

"For, each anatomical structure, each atom, each vibration of each organ, must be able to rebuild itself--if there will be the returning of the elements for its recuperation to any extent. There must be created--in mind, in purpose, in body--those influences and forces that will resuscitate life itself in each cellular unit of the body.
"These activities must begin within self as for a purpose, as for hope, as for desire. Not as boastful, not as egotistical, but that each word, each act, each hope, each element of activity, is to be selfless and unto the glory of Creative Forces, or God." 2994-1

CHAPTER TWENTY-THREE

RELAXATION AND MEDITATION

Under the strain of work-a-day hurry and worry, the nerve vibrations are apt to become more and more intense and excited. They run away with you until, as the saying goes, "you are flying all to pieces."

A good illustration for this condition of the nervous system may be found in a team of horses shying at some object in their path. The driver, panic-stricken has dropped the reins, the frightened horses have taken the bits between their teeth and are dashing headlong down the road, until their master regains control, checks the animals in their maddened course, and compels them to resume their ordinary pace.

So, the high-strung, over-sensitive individual, must gain control over his nervous system, and must subdue his own runaway mental and emotional activities into restful, harmonious vibrations.

This is done by insuring sufficient rest and sleep under ideal conditions, and by practicing relaxation and meditation.

> "Concentration upon relaxation is the greater or better manner for any body to relax. That is, see the body relaxing, consciously...let all of the tension, all of the strain, flow out of self--and find the body giving, giving away."
>
> 404-5
>
> "Q.- What can I do to ease my nervous condition?
> "A.- Relaxing of the body at regular periods is the best. This is much better than depending upon outside influences. Extra amounts of B_1 vitamin will be the better way and manner of booster, but perfect relaxation is the best remedy. Have a period when you forget everything. Not necessarily having to go to sleep to do so; but if you go to sleep during those

periods this is very well. But let the recupe-
ration come from deep within self." 3120-2

"There should not be an overtaxing of the body;
and there should be periods of relaxation, as
there must be in everyone's experience."
                                                        1334-2
Therefore:

"Mentally and physically there should be
relaxation for the body for the best mental,
physical and material development." 2597-2

Meditation:

"Q.- How can I overcome the nerve strain I'm
under at times?
"A.- By closing the eyes and meditating from
within, so that there arises--through that of
the nerve system--that necessary element that
makes along the pineal (don't forget that this
runs from the toes to the crown of the head!)
that will quiet the whole nerve forces, making
for that--as has been given--as the true bread,
the true strength of life itself. Quiet,
meditation, for a half to a minute, will bring
strength--will the body see physically this
flowing out to quiet self, whether walking,
standing still, or resting. Well, too, that
oft when alone, meditate in the silence--as
the body has done." 311-4

Therefore:

"Meditation is emptying self of all that
hinders the creative forces from rising along
the natural channels of the physical man to
be disseminated through those centers and
sources that create the activities of the
physical, the mental, the spiritual man;
properly done must make one stronger mentally,
physically for has it not been given He went

*in the strength of that meat received for many
days? Was it not given by Him who has shown
us the Way, "I have had meat that ye know not
of"? As we give out, so does the whole of man
--physically and mentally--become depleted,
yet in entering into the silence, entering
into the silence of meditation, with a clean
hand, a clean body, a clean mind, we may
receive that strength and power that fits each
individual, each soul, for a greater activity
in this material world."* 281-13

Usually, the victim of unbalanced nerves is of
the high-strung, sensitive type, naturally inclining
to more rapid vibrations on all planes, capable of
much greater achievement than the stolid, heavy, slow-
vibrating person who does not know that he has any
nerves, but also is in greater danger of mental and
emotional overstrain and physical depletion as a result
of the excessive and uncontrolled expenditure of life
force and nervous energy.

At first glance this expression may seem paradox-
ical, but experience will teach that it is not only
possible, but absolutely necessary that we perform our
work in a relaxed and serene condition of body and
mind. The most strenuous physical and mental labor
will then not cause as much exhaustion as light work
done in a state of nervous tension, irritability,
fretfulness, or worry.

Relaxation while working necessitates plan and
system. Most nervous break-downs results not so much
from overwork as from the vitality being wasted through
lack or orderly and harmonious procedures.

Therefore, take some time to plan and arrange your
work, and form the habit of doing certain things that
have to be done every day as nearly as possible, in
the same way (making sure that it is the right way), at
the same time each day. Such an orderly system will
soon become habitual, and result in saving a lot of
valuable time and energy. The same may be said for a
period set aside for meditation, it must be done at
the same time and place each and every day.

*"Through the thorough application of mind over
the existent condition and with the application
of that that will assist, both physical and
mental, in bringing that condition about, from
a physical viewpoint. That is, by this constant entering in, at a specific time, the
quietude of self, or into the silence with
self, for at least--beginning first for five
to ten minutes, increasing this, day by day,
a few minutes, until at least thirty minutes
may be spent in such." 4239-1*

*"Q.- Where shall this body take this solitude,
when concentrating?*
*"A.- Any place the body may choose, being
alone, and in the same place each day."137-3*

*"Q.- What is the best time for meditation for
this entity?*
*"A.- Whenever there is the call, as it were, to
prayer, to service, to aid another. Preferably
in those hours when there is quiet, either in
the evening or the early morning hours."*
                                                    275-39

Additionally, do always cultivate a serene and
cheerful attitude of mind and soul, taking whatever
comes as a part of the day's lessons doing the best
under the cicumstances, but absolutely refusing, to
worry and fret about anything. Not crossing a bridge
before reaching it, nor wasting time.

MEDITATION WHILE SITTING

Sit upright in a comfortable chair without any
strain or tension, spine and head erect and straight,
legs forming right angles with the thighs (the chair
should be neither too high nor too low), feet resting
firmly on the floor, toes pointing slightly outward,
the forearms resting lightly upon the legs with the
hands facing up upon the knees. This must be accomplished without effort, for effort means tension.
Dismiss all thoughts of hurry, care, worry, fear,

etc., and dwell instead upon the following thoughts:

"I am now completely relaxed in body and mind. I am receptive to nature's harmonious, invigorating, vibrations, they dispel the discordant and destructive vibrations of hurry, worry, fear, and anger. New life, new health, new strength are entering into me with every breath, pervading my whole being."

Repeat these thoughts mentally, or, if it helps, say them aloud several times over, quietly and forcefully, impressing them deeply upon your inner consciousness. The follow this with a short period of quiet meditation and contemplation.

> *"Meditate oft. Separate thyself for a season from the cares of the world. Get close to nature and learn from the lowliest of that which manifests in nature, in the earth; in the birds, in the trees, in the grasses, in the flowers, in the bees; that the life of each is a manifestation, is a song of glory to its Maker. And do thou likewise." 1089-3*

Therefore:

> *"In the developing, then, that the man may be one with the Father, necessary that the soul, with its companion the will, through all the various stages of development, until the will is lost in Him and he becomes one with the Father." 900-10*

So in the battle of life, the more faith we have in God, in ourselves, and in our own powers, the wider we open ourselves to the inflow of wisdom and strength from all that is good and true and powerful in the universe. But through persistent and well directed effort only can we control the powers and fashion the materials which nature has so lavishly bestowed upon all of us.

The creative will, actuated by desire and enlightened by reason, brings order and harmony out of chaotic forces and materials. And yet certain metaphysicians tell us that we ourselves must do nothing to overcome weakness, sin and suffering, and that we must depend entirely upon the efficiency of metaphysical formulas, that the diety and the powers of nature are jealous of our personal efforts, that we must not try to help ourselves lest we forfeit their good will.

Is it not blasphemous to assume that God would blame us and withhold his help because we dared use the faculties, capacities, and powers with which He has endowed upon us." You say that, "Nobody is foolish enough to claim such things." But this is the teaching of some healing cults. Its members are forbidden, on penalty of expulsion, to use in the treatment of human ailments the most innocent of natural remedies. The giving of a colonic, or the common-sense regulation of diets are regarded as sufficient to so nullify the power of their metaphysical formulas and to prevent the working of nature's healing forces.

Amidst all the extremes, the methods of natural healing points to the common sense middle way. Basing its teachings and practices on a clear understanding of the laws of health, disease, and cure, it refrains from suppressing acute diseases with poisonous drugs realizing that they are in reality nature's cleansing and healing efforts. Neither does it sit idly by and expect the Lord or metaphysical formulas, or drugs to do our work and to make good for our violations of the laws of nature.

Understanding the law, is then cooperating with the law; is giving the Lord a helping hand. It teaches that "God helps him who helps himself," that He will not become angry and refuse His help if His children use wrongly the reason, the will-power, and the self-control with which he has endowed them, so that they may achieve their own salvation.

The methods of natural healing is but one great prayer from beginning to end. It teaches the law on all planes of being, the physical, the mental, the moral, and the spiritual; and it insists that the only way to attain perfect health of body, mind, and soul is to comply with the law to the best of our ability.

When this is done, we place ourselves in align-

ment, in attunement with the constructive principles
existing in nature, and in exact proportion with the
obedience to the laws of our being, all good things,
the abundance, will come to us. However:

> "...let the policies, the purposes, be not
> alone for the material gain. For remember,
> these should be ever secondary. While it is
> true that in a material world the material
> things are necessities for material activities,
> if the promptings of the activities are of a
> CONSTRUCTIVE nature, God--or the Creative
> Force, or the Divine--gives the increase.
> "For man may not do other than be the channel
> through which the increase of ANY nature may
> arise. For God alone gives the increase.
> "Then, in such an association, with those acti-
> vities, we may bring, we may expect results.
> "And if you do not expect, how CAN it be cre-
> ative? For the increase in material things,
> in the activities that are necessary to be
> increased to meet that need that would CONTINUE
> for the soul development?
> "For the purposes of each entity, each soul,
> in a manifested experience, should ever be to
> do whatever is necessary for the full awaken-
> ing of the purpose that the Creative Force or
> God, or the Universal Energy (or whatever term
> may be necessary for the individual awakening)
> might be expressed.
> "For only with the purpose held in that direc-
> tion may there be the vision of the glory that
> is prepared for those who seek to know His Face.
> "Use the abilities, then, in the direction that
> has been awakened so oft; that alone has kept
> the EFFORTS OF THE ENTITY as a growing experi-
> ence. For know that only as we sow do we reap.
> "As you then sow CONSTRUCTIVE influences into
> the lives and experiences of others, you make
> such growth in your OWN relationships to the
> WHOLE." 1463-1

CHAPTER TWENTY-FOUR

HOW SHALL WE PRAY

Shall we say: "Father, give me this!"---"Father, do for me that!" Or shall we say: "Behold, I am perfect! Imperfection, sin, and suffering, are only errors of mortal mind!"

Or shall we pray: "Father, give me of Thy strength that I may live in harmony with Thy law, for thus only then will all good come to me."

The first way is to beg; the second, to steal; and the third, to earn by honest effort.

"Father give me this!"---"Father do for me that!" Thus doing, our earthly fathers, not understanding, that the great law of compensation, the law of giving and receiving, demands that we give an equivalent for for everything that we receive. Who receives without giving is a beggar.

> "In giving one attains. In giving one acquires. In giving, love comes as the fulfillment of desire, guided, directed, in the ways that bring the more perfect knowledge of application of self as related to the universal, all powerful, all guiding, all divine influence in in life--or it is life." 345-1

The lily, in return for the nourishment that it receives from the soil and the sun, gives its beauty and fragrance. The birds of the air give a return for their sustenance by their songs, the beauty of their plumage, and by destroying insects, the enemies of plant and man.

Every living thing gives an equivalent for its existence in some way or another.

With man, the fulfillment of the law of service and of compensation becomes conscious and voluntary, and his self-respect refuses to take without giving.

379

*"For in the beauty of service comes the know-
ledge and the understanding that makes the
living worthwhile. Setting aside those things
that so easily beset, looking forward to that
mark of that higher calling as is set in Him,
knowing that the greatest service that may be
done is the little word here and there, the
kindly thought, the little deeds that make the
heart glad, and the brightness of the Son come
in the lives of all." 262-13*

"Behold I am perfect! Imperfection, as sin and
suffering are only errors of mortal mind!" Such is the
prayer of certain metaphysical healers.

To assume the possession of goodness and perfection without an earnest effort to develop and to deserve
these qualities means to steal the glory of the Perfect
One. The assumption of present perfection precludes the
necessity of striving and laboring for its attainment.
If I am already all goodness, all love, all wisdom,
and all power, what remains for me to strive for?

Herein lies the danger of metaphysical idealism.
While it may dispel pessimism, fear, and anxiety, it
inevitably weakens the will-power and the capacity to
help one's self through one's own personal efforts.

The ideal of the metaphysician is the ideal of
the animal. The animal does not worry about right or
wrong, nor with few exceptions, does it make provision
for the future. Its care and forethought extend only
to the next meal. But this perfect, ideal, passive
trust in nature's bounty causes the animal to remain
animal and prevents its rising above the narrow limitations of habit and instinct.

The inherent faculties, capacities, and powers of
the human soul can be developed only by effort and use.
The savage, living in the most favored regions of the
earth, depending for his sustenance in perfect faith
and trust on nature's never-failing bounty, has ever
remained savage. Through ages he has risen but little
above the level of the beast, that lives, eats and then
perishes.

The great law of use ordains that those faculties

and powers which we do not develop remain in abeyance,
and that those which we possess weaken and atrophy if
we fail to exercise them.

The Master Jesus emphasized this law of usage in
many of his parables and sayings.

"For whosoever hath, to him shall be given, and
he shall have more abundance: but whosoever hath not,
from him shall be taken away even that he hath."

What does this mean? Those who have the desire
and the will to work out their own salvation, acquire
greater knowledge and power in exact proportion to
their well directed efforts; but those who have neither
the desire nor the will to help themselves, lose their
natural endowments and the possibilities and opportunities which these would have conferred upon them.

> *"For, no soul or entity enters without opportu-*
> *nities. And the choice is ever latent within*
> *self and the power, the ability to do things, be*
> *things, to accept things, is with the entity."*
> 3226-1
>
> *"Then, use thy opportunities--not as privileges*
> *of abuse, but opportunities for service. For,*
> *"He that is the greatest among you is servant*
> *of all" said He who is the way, the truth, the*
> *light to all." 2251-1*

Therefore:

> *"Opportunities present themselves each day.*
> *For as has been just been given, it is not by*
> *other than growth that there are the greater*
> *opportunities or activities of the body with*
> *an organization of such broad activity."*
> 1120-3

And:

> *Opportunities are expressions of appreciation*
> *from thy Maker. Embrace them--not for self but*
> *for the glory of thy Maker." 2051-5*

The anatomy and physiology of the human brain
reveal the fact that for every voluntary faculty,
capacity, and power of body, mind, and soul which we
wish to develop, we have to energize new cells and
centers in the brain. In this respect, nature gives
us no more and no less than what we deserve and work
for. If we "try to cheat" by ursurping the perfection
and the power which we have not honestly earned and
developed, then sometimes, somewhere we shall have to
square the balance.

After all the only true prayer is personal effort
and self-help. This does not mean that we should not
invoke the help of our Higher Powers, but we should
pray for strength to do our work, and not to have it
done for us, thereby shirking our responsibilities.
The wise parent will not do for the child the home
tasks assigned him at school. Neither will the powers
from on High or the Father perform our alloted tasks
for us. Not by any means.

This life is a schoolhouse for personal effort.
If it were not so, life would be meaningless. From
the cradle to the grave, our days are one continuous
effort to learn, to acquire, to overcome all diffi-
culties. Only in this way can we develop our latent
faculties, capacities and strengths. These cannot be
developed by having our task done for us, nor by the
assumption that we already know and possess all that
we will ever need or have need for.

The athlete must do his own training. No one else
can do it for him. The assumption of superiority over
his opponent will not develop his suppleness of body
and strength of muscle. To be sure, faith and courage
are essential to victory, but they must be backed by
careful and persistent training. Vainglorious boasting will not win the contest, ever.

> *"When one develops muscle and brawn for the
> ring, or for any activity of such nature, there
> are certain rules of living that must be
> adhered to, or that have been found to be
> necessary for such an one to adhere to.*
> *"When a faculty of the body, as a pianist, or*

cornetist, or an artist, is to be developed,
there are certain courses of development, cer-
tain training through which the body-physical,
the body-mental, shall pass as training self
for such an undertaking.
"When one, then, is to develop a faculty, or
a force, that is present--as any of these
referred to, lying latent in one form or
another in every individual; so, then, do the
psychic forces, the psychic faculties, lie
dormant or active in every individual, and
await only that awakening or arousing, or the
developing under those environs that make for
the accentuation of same in the individual."
5752-1
"That which is in keeping with the law of
Creative Forces, or energies, is developing.
That which is of self, self-aggrandizement,
self-indulgence alone, is retarding." 2329-1

Therefore:

"As the activities of self are expressed in
that done unto others, so is the abundance of
love, companionship, expression of His close-
ness, found in thine experience." 262-51

Therefore we pray: "Father, give me of Thy strength
that I may live in harmony with thy Law, for thus only
will all good come to me."

"For, from the abundance of the heart the mouth
speaketh truth." 262-51

Leaving the main thread of our lessons and coming into the personal life of each student who is following this line of investigation, we offer a few remarks merely as advice and not as instruction.

In the first place every owner of this volume who pursues its studies in a scholarly manner, is regarded as a student. But this means and requires more than reading and re-reading its pages. A true student applies and makes notes and preserves facts of experiences, whether they came to him through other channels, or by reason of his own investigations and experiments. He, therefore, will deal with a volume of this character as if it were a teacher talking to him and working with him in the privacy of his home. He will preserve all the data that may fall to him, for future reference and study.

This study is a most useful branch of education in life that will be extremely beneficial, fitting us adequately for actual contact with the mundane world. As years roll by and the new influences accumulate and enlarge into one vast field of experience, as an ever increasing love for the periods devoted to this self-education will ever draw us to the pages of this book which we have now closed. No historic college walls can furnish grander environments, and no Alma Mater sweeter memories than the places and hours devoted to the unfolding of a new life and a personal power but which may laid hidden forever if not awakened.

A growth that is real is not noticeable day by day. True progress must have an inward beginning and an outward unfolding. Growth that is visible is mere bloating of the ego. Beware of the latter. When you have graduated from the eleventh stage, if the work has been faithfully done, you will have made all the progress that should be achieved. The perpetual regime will keep you ever growing and increasing, year by year, until no person is your superior in well-being and personal power.

THE END